To Jada
With Love &
Vijay

Unfolding
Happiness

Ambika Devi, MA

&

Vijay Jain, MD

Unfolding Happiness

Ambika Devi, MA

&

Vijay Jain, MD

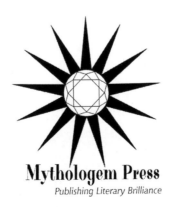

Mythologem Press
Publishing Literary Brilliance

For information contact:
Mythologem Press
www.MythologemPress.com
VOX 772-233-8229
MythologemPress@gmail.com
www.UnfoldingHappiness.com

FIRST EDITION

Designed by Ambika Devi, MA and Ron Birchenough
Cover art by Ambika Devi, MA
Vintage images

Library of Congress Catalog-in-Publication Data
Ford, Amy a.k.a. Ambika Devi, MA 1959-
Jain, Vijay 1947-
ISBN-13: 978-0-9978678-1-7
ISBN-10: 0-9978678-1-7

Entire manuscript completed November 25, 2015, 11:21:36 p.m.

Printed in the United States of America

MEDICAL DISCLAIMER
This book does not provide medical advice; its content and suggestions do not substitute for consultation with a physician. Medical and nutritional sciences change rapidly, and information contained in this book may not be current when read. Neither the publisher nor the authors are liable for any loss, injury, or damage arising from information in this book, including loss or injury from typographical errors.

A Blessing for All

Lord with the elephant face, served by all the Ganas, who takes as his food,

the essence of kapitta and jambuphala (two favorite fruits of Ganesha),

Son of Uma (Parashakti) he who is destroyer of sorrow and remover of obstacles,

we worship at your divine Lotus Feet.

In deep gratitude I honor Lord Ganesha,

guardian of the gate that leads to Mother.

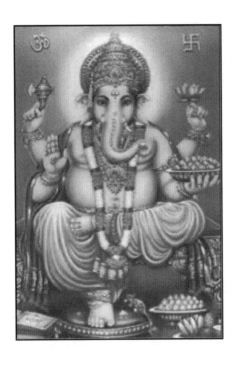

।। श्री गणेश शलोक: ।।

गजाननम् भूत गणादि सेवितम्

GajAnanaM BhUta GaNAdhi sevitaM

कपित्थ जम्बू फल सार भक्षितम्

kapittha jambU phala sAra Baxitam

उमा सुतम् शोक विनाश कारकम्

umA sutaM shoka vinAsha kArakam

नमामि विघ्नेश्वर पाद पङ्कजम्

namAmi vighneshvara pAda paÑkajam

I salute unto the Lord, Vasudeva, the Master of Time,

and offer myself to Lord Dhanvantari, the Master of Medicine,

who holds the pot of nectar that destroys all illnesses,

and who is the Master of the Three Worlds

and the Protector of the Universe.

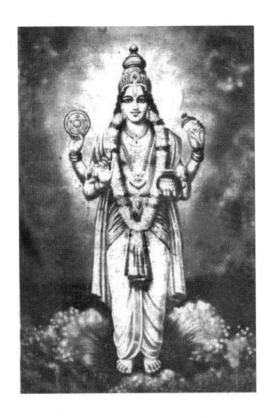

ॐ नमो भगवते वासुदेवाय

AUM namo Bhagavte vAsudevAya

धनवन्तरये अमृतकलशहसताय

Dhanvantaraye amR^itakalashastrAya

सर्वामयविनशाय त्रैलोक्यनाथाय

sarvAmayavinashAya TrailokyanAthAya

श्री महविष्णवे स्वाहा

shrI mahAviShNave svAha

DEDICATION

We are grateful for the blessing of Ganesha and appreciatively dedicate the offering of this writing to Sri Dhanvantari and you kind readers. May all who drink in these words find happiness.

With love, Ambika and Vijay

TABLE OF CONTENTS

Unfolding Happiness

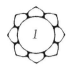

INTRODUCTION

Happiness becomes our true nature once we learn to let go of anything that gets in the way of sharing love. We are spiritual beings having human experiences, and the primary purpose of our mission is to share love. The Dalai Lama teaches that we feel happy when we are happy for another's happiness. This understanding reveals the possibility of living life as a vibrant and joyous celebration.

The state of happiness can be elusive. We cannot create it, but we can remove the obstacles that hide it from our perception. In this way we are able to skillfully unfold seeming obstructions to reveal our capacity to be in a truly happy state of being.

Happiness is the greatest prosperity we can experience. It goes far beyond the idea of material wealth. When we reach a state—and it is a state—of happiness, the desire to prove to others why we are happy disappears. The thoughts and stories we share in this book are ideas and tools of self-discovery we have found along our personal paths. They have lifted the veil and helped to unfold and reveal happiness as a real place of being. They are our experiences. It is our hope that we can help you, dear reader, in your search for happiness.

The title of our book, "Unfolding Happiness," was inspired by a lotus seed that gestates, grows and unfolds into a beautiful lotus flower, revealing its splendor and true nature. Under favorable circumstances, the seeds of the lotus can remain viable for centuries. The oldest recorded lotus seed to germinate is from a 1,300 year old specimen that was recovered from a dry lakebed in northeastern China.

The patience of the lotus seed inspires us to know that it does not matter how long the journey to unfold our true nature of happiness takes. Just as the flower's full potential is held within the seed, so is our own possibility. It just needs to be nurtured and then, by its true nature, unfolds when the conditions are right.

Throughout history, the image of a lotus flower has often been used as an example of divine beauty. Every part and stage of its development holds significant meaning. The seed represents potential. The stem illustrates a connection between water, earth, and sky, and relates to our bodies, minds, and spirits in this way. In Hindu art, the thrones and pedestals used in the creative expression of the gods is often the blossom of a lotus flower. In its fully open form, it also represents the Sun, the supporter of life on our planet and the center of our solar system. The Hindu deity Vishnu, often referred to as the "Lotus-Eyed One," signifies the sustainer of the universe.

The image of a lotus flower's unfolding petals suggests the expansion of the soul. The growth of its pure beauty from the muck and mud of its origin holds a spiritual promise of revealing its true nature. A Confucian scholar, Zhou Dunyi, wrote, "I love the lotus because while growing from mud, it is unstained."

Here we share our ideas and feelings about the unfolding of happiness, classified in distinct chapters that relate to the phases of the lotus flower's life and regeneration cycle. We invite you to think of the entirety of this book as an ongoing process in which all the information is a continuum that merges into itself.

Enjoy the journey from identifying the seed that carries the potential of happiness—through the nourishment stage where we explore the creation of a nurturing environment for the seeds of happiness to unfold, grow, and flourish. We encourage you to try the ideas and offerings that we share and hope they lead you to a happy life filled with joy and bliss.

Gratefully, Ambika Devi, MA and Vijay Jain, MD

SEED
The potential of happiness is found in meditation

We all want to be happy. In fact, happiness is our true nature. Happiness is a constant, like Primordial Energy. It is always there, like the sun, which is always shining. Sometimes clouds block the view, but when the wind blows or the heat of the sun's rays dissolves the obstruction, we see and feel its light shining once again. The flow of life in an effortless, graceful manner is our birthright. Life is supposed to be without struggle.

To be in a state of happiness is unique and individual. It can be quickly triggered and affected by things, places, and events. Even though happiness is our true nature, some people are happy while others are not. Happiness becomes obscure when we forget that it is a state of being rather than something we create by means of outside sources. It is like the tight bud of a flower that needs to be urged to unfold with tenderness and love.

Many factors can interrupt the process of our opening. Society and the external world fool us into believing an ideal of what "perfect" is supposed to look like and what happiness should be. As we observe the world around us, we notice that some people seem to be happy regardless of their situation, while others are challenged to be happy no matter how perfect their lives appear on the surface.

The media and ideas easily trick us into believing that we can find true and lasting happiness through material trappings. The pressures we experience confuse us and disguise the pathway to happiness. Our attachment to an ideal body image can lead us to a path of manipulation, often placing the body at risk and creating a perception of unhappiness.

When we engage in further self-study and dial our inner vision into focus, we are able to clearly see that the objects and situations we initially desired ultimately become the source of misery. It is due to these vestiges of living that the attainment of happiness can easily elude us. Rather than thinking about what happiness is supposed to be, what we really need is to be taught to identify what happiness feels like.

To increase our potential level of happiness, it is important to partake in daily practices that help to remind us that we are always connected to a greater energy. This in turn helps us to be in a continual state of trust. Here we find it easier to accept the present and place less importance on a perception of what is right or wrong.

All it takes in any given moment is a small, simple, little suggestion. Say you are out walking on a path, there are people passing you on bicycles, your phone rings, and for a split second you sense your morning walk is creating stress rather than peace and solitude.

What if you stop and ask your mind, "Can we be still and quiet for just a moment?"

Here is something you can try:

Stop whatever you are doing. Turn your phone off for a few minutes and free your arms. Perhaps jump up and down and let the body shake out in no particular way. Maybe your voice wants to make noise.

Now stand where you are and become perfectly still. Close your eyes. Connect to the vastness of infinite space. Instantaneously you are able to tune into the sounds of birds and insects. Feel the sensation of the air upon your skin. Notice the moisture within the mouth and the taste of the saliva. Let the smell of earth and flowers dance in your nostrils.

What does the environment sound like now? What does the expression on your face feel like? Just be absolutely still and see where this takes you. Perhaps the body begins to move and dance or shake. Maybe you will yell or cry or smile. There is no right or wrong. This is an opportunity to let go of the mind and just observe, as if you are viewing someone else.

Once you find yourself still again, tune into your breath and perhaps even your heart beating. In the silent spaces at the top of your breath when the lungs fill to capacity, do you notice any sensation? At the bottom of your breath when the belly draws in, what are you feeling?

Slowly open the eyes and begin to take in the environment surrounding you. At first there is just a little light seeping into your awareness. Then, as the eyelids gently open, you are greeted with a flood of shapes and colors. Notice how the light of the sun brightens the hues of the plants and trees, and how in this moment there is beauty in you and everything around you. What are the sensations?

This is a very humble yoga[1] exercise that tunes us into the wisdom of Ayurveda[2]. This simple practice is a taste of meditation. By bringing our awareness to a focal point, it shows us our ability to be in the present moment. This in turn points out that everything we need to feel good and to be happy is already inside of us.

The qualities of these impressions determine the quality of our thoughts and feelings. We experience the world through the five sensory organs attached to our corresponding senses all at the physical level of our being. These same senses and sensory organs are also associated with five elements and five motor organs.

Here is something you can try:

Try experiencing the cosmic components of the universe. Begin with a morning walk before sunrise. Look into the sky and take in the elements of space, with stars twinkling. Notice how the sounds of nature are abundant at this time of the day and how the chorus of birds begins to sing. If you are near water, listen to the changes in the sound of it,

---

1 **Yoga** योग *yoga* A physical, mental and spiritual discipline originating in ancient India.
2 **Ayurveda** आयुर्वेद *Ayurveda* Ayurveda is the traditional healing modality of the Vedic culture from India, said to be 2000 to 5000 years old. Ayurveda literally translates as "the wisdom of life" or "the knowledge of longevity."

whether you are at the shore and hearing waves crashing, or by a creek listening to the trickling sound dancing across stones or pebbles. What does the morning air feel and taste like? When the sun begins to appear, it fills the vast emptiness of space with the fire element rising in the sky. Feeling the warmth of sun on the body, coupled with sound of water and earth underfoot, completes the full sensory experience.

A little story

To explain this, we wish to share a little story about a financial advisor who was on vacation in the Caribbean. There he sat on a gorgeous white beach, gazing out on turquoise water ordering fruity drinks.

A tanned, young cabana boy no more than eleven years old dutifully brought the beverages. Palm trees gently swayed and cooled the man in their striated shadows. Peaceful waves rolled in and out as sunlight danced on the water.

After the third round of tropical coolers, the man called the boy over and asked him, "Do you go to school?"

"No," said the boy with a wide smile.

"Don't you want to go to school?" the man asked.

"Why?" replied the boy, twirling his toes in the sand. "What would that do?"

"You could be educated and then get a job," said the man with a smirk.

"What would that do?" the boy asked, watching the clouds change shape over head.

"You could get a job, make money" was the reply.

The boy's forehead wrinkled slightly as he looked directly in the eyes of the man. Upon seeing his confusion, the man continued.

"With more money, you could go on vacation." Still the boy did not seem convinced. This inspired the man to continue. "Then you could be happy."

The boy's face lit up in a huge gleaming smile. The man thought he had hit the jackpot, but the boy responded, "Why would I do that? I am already happy!" he laughed.

The external successes of wealth, possessions, and status are put upon us by society. People who are able to live closer to nature are more at peace with their surroundings and experience a higher level of happiness.

It is a known fact that the greater number of happy people fall into what the masses of society would classify as a lower income bracket. We must look at the statistical information regarding external successes, wealth, and partnerships that blast our senses through the media. These are not at all necessary for us to find happiness.

Our individual disposition is based on the unique inherited imprint of our psycho-physical constitution. We come into this world, and our families, to find gifts and obstacles along our path. These present us with opportunities and pose challenges. It is up to us how we react to them. The example of the cabana boy on the beach shows a clear connection to the present moment and the mind projections that a vacationer can easily have.

Our spirit is part of a unified field of consciousness. It remains a constant. The primitive mind functions as a servant; it performs the tasks of bringing in information and energy through our senses that our consciousness, intellect, and ego want us to believe, and then transports these qualities into the body. The purpose of sensory experiences is for sustaining the physical body and mind. When we use our senses excessively, we take on too much of these experiences and store them. This is difficult to metabolize. Undigested reality then remains in our physiology and acts as a toxin. Eventually, this leads to disease and unhappiness. Bringing in the right amount of sensory input, at the right time, is intuitive and automatic if we are able to listen to our higher self. The body is the end result of our sensory experiences that have been metabolized in the linear past. Changing the body occurs when we shift our perceptions of experiences.

We were walking and chatting one morning discussing these ideas. "Do you feel you learned this in your elementary school?" Ambika asked. She had a hunch that Vijay's foundational healing magic went back much further than medical school.

Here is the story that he shared about his early experience at the J.P. Adarsh School with his first teacher, J.P. Singh, in Delhi, India.

"My first formal education experience was in a one-room neighborhood school when I was five years old. My parents chose this for me due to the close proximity to our home, which allowed me to join my mother each afternoon for lunch. In addition, they felt strongly about the fact that my teacher, Mr. J.P. Singh, began each morning with an hour-long spiritual discourse. My parents believed this would instill a strong sense of duty and responsibility in me and would teach me to honor my family and society as well as lay an integral foundation stone of trust in a higher power.

"The comfortable, open classroom was the ground floor of my teacher's house right next door to my family's home. Twenty of us, ranging from myself at five years of age to the eldest of eleven, were in attendance. This blending of grades one through five created a sense of brother and sisterhood.

"The initial lesson I learned was that the first child to arrive each morning was assigned the task of being the monitor for the day. Being the daily monitor had responsibilities as well as perks. The duties of the monitor included sweeping the one-room school and seeing that everything was tidy. In addition, during the course of the day the monitor was responsible for maintaining the discipline of classmates, especially when the one and only teacher went on breaks.

"I made up my mind in that moment, in learning of this position, that I would be the monitor every day. Each morning I eagerly awoke at five a.m. and knocked on the door of the school announcing, 'Good morning! This is Vijay from next door. I am the monitor today!'

"'OK!' I would hear the voice of my teacher call from his upstairs quarters.

"I would then return home to ready myself and join my family for breakfast, after which I would return next door to begin my school day.

"Our daily schedule began with an hour of spiritual discourse that was either a reading from the Bhagavad Gita[3] or Ramayana[4]. The morning teaching gave students a thorough understanding of the rights and responsibilities of family and society. We were taught the value of education as the most important possession we could ever obtain. Our teacher instilled in me a strong sense of gratitude for knowledge that has stayed with me throughout this life. In addition, the work ethic of my father and the unconditional love of my mother helped to mold me into a very confident and happy child."

Morals and values are more important than rights. Faith, and subsequently trust, are also important parts of this whole equation. Trust blooms forth from faith, and faith in turn is a result of being in trust. When we experience knowing wisdom, we have an inner sense that we are on the right path. Faith does not require proof. It is a trust that all transformation is the constant pulse of the universe. When we take a leap of faith, we trust that everything is going to be all right.

To our clients and students we can give hope, but they must have faith. Unfolding and subsequently removing obstacles helps us to find our true state of being. Faith gives us the ability to surrender to a higher power. This in turn brings us the confidence that we can indeed grow and get better in any situation.

Vijay shares this story from a visit to India in 2001 to help us understand this further.

"I am sitting in my sister's car and she is driving. We come to an intersection at a traffic light. As we stop at the light, a kid not more than six years old comes to the passenger side of the car and asks for money, pointing to his empty belly. He is dressed in rags and has not taken a bath in several days. He looks sad as he continues his request. My sister shouts from the driver seat, instructing me not to give the boy any money. The

---

3 **Bhagavad Gita** भगवद्गीता *bhagavadgItA* A 700-verse Hindu scripture that is part of the epic Mahabharata. It is classified as स्मृति *smriti* and Krishna's song.
4 **Ramayana** रामायण *rAmAyana* An ancient epic written in Sanskrit depicting the journey of राम *Rama*, considered to be the seventh avatar of विष्णु *Vishnu*, the all preserving essence of all beings in the Trimurti.

child then runs away to the sidewalk as the light turns green. I see him laughing with other kids who are also begging. Where did his hunger go, I wonder? Was he really sad or just acting? He is totally unaffected by his role and gets back to his real self once he is not performing. He seems happy doing what kids do and is able to distance himself from his acting role."

What about us as adults? We are so fused with our roles that we think we are the parts we are playing. We forget who we are at our core. We lose track of consciousness and the "I," which is unaffected by the characters we are playing. It is when we surrender and become a witness to all of this that true happiness is experienced, like that of the child on the street.

Primordial Energy

Primordial energy is the animating force that is the womb of all creation. It is not tangible to the senses. When condensed, it appears in the form of light; when it is further condensed, it appears in the form of matter. All of the gross elements and everything in nature come from primordial energy and therefore it can seem to have magical qualities.

What we truly are is a part of the infinite space of primordial energy. The four elements of Air, Fire, Water, and Earth come from the element of Space. What sets Space apart from the other four is that it is a constant. It can never decompose; the other four can.

When we realize what we are made of and how we fit in to the greater scheme of things, we feel connected to all that is. This makes us feel happy. The teachings of Yoga are geared at bringing us into this awareness through the modality of meditation. It is in the meditative state that we find our true beingness, our own infinite space. When we are in touch with this, we are happy.

To increase our potential level of happiness, it is important to partake in daily practices that help to remind us that we are always connected to a greater energy. This in turn helps us to be in a continual state of trust. In this place we find it easier to accept the present moment and place less importance on a perception of what is right or wrong.

Traditional Yoga philosophy teaches that we should "become the witness to the modifications of the mind." A great teacher of yoga, Swami Vivekananda, explained to seekers, "The mind behaves like a drunken monkey that has been stung by a scorpion." The celebrated Swami humorously taught that in order to pacify it, "we must give the monkey a banana!" In the teaching of meditation, the "banana" is a sound, a mantra[5]. These primordial sounds tune us into nature and return us to our pure state of being. The science of mantra is very specific to each individual and must be prescribed by an experienced teacher. Factors of birth, location, and timing are all used. Pronunciation is of the utmost importance and, as Ambika's teacher says, "Even a computer refuses to start with an incorrect password." It is also possible to enter this state of being by simply tuning into the breath.

Meditation is a place where we step out of the thinking mind and experience a feeling of disappearing, a deep trance state where we lose track of our edges. These edges are the mind's attachment to the idea that the physical body is who we are. In the meditative state, we realize that the body is a flesh-robe that we wear and that our true state of being is infinite.

There are many pathways into the state of meditation, and three distinct levels. Many of us experience the first stage of finding deep relaxation after physical exertion. This is the "zone" spoken about by so many athletes when hitting their stride, either in competition or a personal workout. Modern culture is now popularizing guided meditation; this integrative state of relaxation is the second level. The third level is the timeless deep trance state of being.

The true meditative state gives us the ability to harmonize and integrate the physical, emotional, intellectual, and spiritual aspects of our existence. In the deep trance state of meditation we disarm the

---

5 Mantra मन्त्र *mantra* A sound, a syllable, a word or group of words possessing transformative power. The words and use are particular to each school of thought and sacred lineage.

voice of the thoughts and the mind. This is the true practice of Yoga, in which we are able to become a witness to the modifications of the mind. The restlessness of the three levels of the mind is what the great sage Patanjali[6] calls Chitta[7] in his famous sutra, "Yoga Chitta Vritti Nirodha[8]." This means that the practice of yoga helps us to become a witness to mind-wave disturbances. The true meditative state gives us the ability to harmonize and integrate the physical, emotional, intellectual, and spiritual aspects of our existence.

In a state of meditation, the mind is like a still and gentle lake—glassy and peaceful. Thoughts and ideas are like a boat that powers against the current. These produce a series of waves that blast to the shoreline. We can get caught in the waves and be tossed onto an unknown shore, we can be sucked under and feel like we are drowning, or we can sit quietly in amazement watching the waves and their wakes of thought. To be in a state of meditation is to simply notice rather than react to all of this. It is human nature to have an initial reaction. Perhaps we first desire to ride the boat, which could lead to wanting to travel out of an uncomfortable current situation. Maybe we become frustrated with the disruption of what was still and glassy just a moment ago and try to race back into the past. Another choice can be to try to ride a particular wave and use force in order to land in a specific place.

Meditation is the subtlest form of human activity that lets us experience the true nature of self. Our true self is the underlying field of pure consciousness and is the state of bliss, optimum health, and happiness. When we are established in this state we don't need external sources to make us happy—we are just happy. Meditation guides us to the realization that everything in the universe is connected. In the state of meditation we can witness an occurrence yet have a full sense of being removed from it. This means we are joyous, content, blissful, and

---

6 **Patanjali** पतञ्जलि *patanjali* Name of a philosopher who was also a physician. He lived 150 BCE.

7 **Chitta** चित्त *citta* Thought.

8 **Yoga Chitta Vritti Nirodha** योग: चित्त वृत्ति निरोध: : *yogaH chitta vR^itti nirodhaH* Yoga is a set of contextual directions to individuals, for the goal of refining and regulating psycho-spiritual propensities.

connected. We are accepting of the present moment as it is without any feeling of needing to change.

Once we are able to easily find our way into a meditative state, we can then walk and function in this condition. Our actions are guided spontaneously to fulfill our needs and our desires according to the laws of nature. Living our life is free of suffering when every thought and action is spontaneously correct. This creates an ease of giving in love and relationships and connecting at deeper levels with all beings.

Meditation is the only way to discover what truth is. Knowledge of truth alone cannot take us to truth. Neither can the practice of feeling the truth. Truth exists beyond the mind. When we live in the spirit of our intellectual convictions, we live in truthfulness. This is how we cultivate a high level of integrity. Direct experience in the practice of meditation is what leads us to a state of truth, bliss, and happiness. In the practice of meditation we go beyond the mind and encounter our true self, which is the witness to everything. In this contemplative state, we recognize and experience the essential blissful nature of self. This is how we find out who we truly are.

Positive effects of a steady meditation practice are a state of profound relaxation, which relieves anxiety, and a canceling of stressors that are known to be the cause of eighty percent of all diseases. In addition, meditation has been found in numerous studies to reverse or slow the aging process.

When we feel connected we are able to spend quality time and share in loving communication with those around us. It becomes easier to see the best in others. Mundane actions like cooking and cleaning become magical. Flavors and colors are enhanced. Vision becomes focused and senses sharpen. Small token gifts, like a flower or a pebble, become sacred.

Many indigenous tribes, like the Hopi, teach their teens the importance of this type of connecting. Young braves spend long hours creating intricate beadwork to decorate themselves in order to attract a mate. This is a form of meditation. In addition, they practice playing the flute, singing, and dancing to show their love. These are vital ways to share life energy and, in this way, their lives are a form of moving meditation.

The same is true when we give fully and freely in our relationships. This offering becomes a sharing of the elements. Loving communication is an expression of space. Hugs, kisses, and touch are the dance of air. When we see the best in others and situations and give genuine compliments, we communicate with the passionate element of fire. Compassion and sharing when we cook together are the flowing element of water. The element of earth gives us support and provides the fertile ground to grow our food. These are integral components that create a state of happiness.

Here is something you can try:

Find a comfortable, quiet place where you can spend a few minutes focusing on your breath. Sit with the back as straight as you are able, either on the edge of a chair or seated on the floor. Close your eyes and become aware of your breath. Notice the sensation of the air moving in and out of the nostrils, particularly the front edges of the nostrils. Imagine at what percentage of your lung capacity you are breathing. It is likely to be forty percent or less of your full capacity. Breathe like this for six to ten breaths. Notice the sensations and feelings this produces.

Now increase your breath to fifty percent and notice an instant feeling of relaxation. Do this for another six to ten breaths.

Next increase the breath to seventy-five percent. Allow yourself to yawn and expel the stale and stagnant energy that has been sitting in the bottoms of the lungs. Continue at seventy-five percent of your capacity for several more breaths.

Now breathe a full one-hundred percent, continuing to breathe in through the nose and out through the nose. Next, begin to pause at the top of the breath, when you are filled with air, and slowly exhale completely. Pause again at the bottom of the breath when you are empty, gently drawing the belly toward the spine. Notice the sensation of stillness and calm during the cessation phases.

Write all of the observations about what you have noticed during each stage of this breathing experience in your journal.

Nourishment
Feed happiness by creating an environment of nurturance and love

The Most Powerful Healer Is Love

After many years of working both as a clinician and a surgical physician, Vijay shares his feelings with me regarding what he believes, which is that the true healer in any situation is love. When asked his opinion as to what it is that truly shifted the progression of patients over the years from disease to health and ultimately happiness, he is the first to admit,

"It is not the medicine, or the surgeries or any of the modifications that were offered, as much as the bottom-line-factor of love."

We were walking in the warm morning sunlight, talking about our early education and experiences within various institutions along these present life-paths.

"Vijay, do you think that it is the bedside manner of a doctor that brings the greatest potential of healing?"

Without skipping a beat he answered, "Absolutely!"

As we walked and talked about the topic that morning I was given the opportunity to witness this exact phenomenon in action. At that very moment, his phone rang. It was an old friend, telling him that a mutual longtime friend of theirs, who had been suffering with breast cancer, was in hospice.

We stopped and Vijay called her immediately. I sat nearby and listened to him speak in a soothing and loving tone of voice. It was not so much the words or the pace of his speech but rather the glowing feeling of love that overwhelmed me. As I quietly observed and soaked in the vibrational sensations of his compassionate conduct, I was moved to tears.

There is a look that goes along with a feeling when we watch another person share from the core of their being. It is different than the sensation of taking in factual knowledge, like that of the study of geography or math. With this type of communication there is an earth-moving feeling. I can only describe it as an awareness that God is speaking to me directly. This is when I can feel the divine primordial power coming clearly through another human being.

It is in a state of love that happiness comes. As I listened to Vijay talk with his friend in the last phase of her present life, I experienced an overwhelming wave of love. It infused every molecule of my being instantaneously. Tears began to trickle from eyes to cheeks, and I had the distinct feeling of love all over and around us. As I observed it, I realized this is not for a person, or a place, or an object, but as a four-year-old once taught me, it is for what he had named "the everything."

After the phone conversation ended, I shared my feelings with Vijay about happiness.

"It is so apparent listening to you speak with your friend that you are full of love," I said. I thought back to the first time I had an appointment with Vijay. I was so sick and had just wanted to give up. I recalled how soothed and safe I felt in his quiet little office in the woods. "The outpouring of love you gave to this patient just now is so overwhelming. Look, it has brought me to tears," I squeaked as I choked a little bit on the emotional wave.

"Well," he began. "She is an old friend. I love her very much."

"I observe you giving this kind of love to everyone," I replied. "This is what I felt instantly when I first came to see you and sought your help. Do you think it is love that heals patients more than anything?" I continued.

"All the advancements in medicine are worthless if they are mechanically dispensed," he stated and went on, "Healing can only come in the presence of love. It is with love that trust is developed in others, and in my case, in patients. I made a decision at one point, when rebuilding my practice, to be accessible and available to everyone who comes to me. This is my way of sharing this love. I am not responsible for the healing. It is my duty only to give love to these individuals."

I continued to feel the warmth of love spread throughout my body as we walked on. I recalled how, just moments ago, while Vijay spoke to his friend that I could sense her energy shift from fear to trust. Though I could not make out the specific words of the conversation, I clearly understood the transference not so much in sound as in sensation. In the flash of a moment I understood that though her soul was in the final phase, facing her step through the ultimate doorway, she was experiencing happiness.

A person does not need to be healthy in order to be happy; happiness is an individual state of mind. Our intellectual point of view can shift in a moment. Our feelings can sail us through daunting situations like thermal currents of air that lift a bird up, allowing it to glide freely. Our state of mind can also cause us to flounder and gasp for air. When we are confused, we become disconnected from what really matters. This is how we buy into illusion which, in turn, leaves us in a state of malcontent.

It is a fact that people who seemingly have very little materially are happier than lottery winners. It is proven that simple pleasures lead us to being blissfully happy. For some reason, it is easier for us to picture a healthy person in a state of true happiness. But what about finding the gift and blessing in a disease. How do we accept the challenges of disease and live in the present moment?

Happiness increases when we feel connected. A daily visit to nature is an important part of linking ourselves to a greater power. According to Ayurveda, that which is in the macrocosm is indeed in the microcosm. This is true of each and every thing in the universe. Stars and planets floating in the infinite space of the cosmos, rocks, plants, trees, and all life-forms are made up of the five gross elemental energies. It is in the experience of our daily visits with nature that we have an opportunity to synchronize with these five elements and get in touch with their presence in everything.

The External World and the Mind

What we experience through sound, touch, sight, taste, and smell has the power to create a sense of happiness by stimulating the production of dopamine and other neurotransmitters including serotonin, oxytocin, and endorphins. These are called "happy chemicals." Through sensory input, these can create a measurable state of happiness. Experiencing the world around us through the five elements of nature—space, air, fire, water, and earth—on a daily basis in their raw forms help to enhance our happiness and help quiet the mind. This helps to take us closer to our true energetic essence.

When we begin to really understand that we are not the ego and stop identifying and getting caught in the web of the roles we play, we really begin to know that we are the unchanging omnipresence. This is when the "I am" becomes established in the self.

Ambika Shares a Story about Learning This through a Simple Saying

"I met Bhante Dharmawara[9] when he was one-hundred-and-three years old. He was a Cambodian-born monk who taught me about meditation, self-acceptance, and peace. Bhante had lived in India for many years and had been a close friend of Gandhi. After being ordained as a Buddhist monk, he moved from India to a monastery in upstate New York. There he met my friend Greg Lynn Weaver, who became his personal attendant.

"Greg Lynn is a fascinating man. He is a healer, a philosopher, a teacher, and a leader. While living in Pennsylvania I had the wonderful pleasure of being a part of his group, 'The Peace Weavers.'

"Prior to my meeting Bhante, Greg Lynn shared many stories about

---

9 **Samdach Vira Dharmawara Bellong Mahathera**, February 12, 1889 – June 26, 1999, also known simply as Bhante Dharmawara by his students, was a Cambodian-born Theravada monk and teacher who died at the age of 110.

the monk and the wisdom of his teachings with our community. We learned that Bhante had attended the Sorbonne in Paris, worked as a magistrate, and played music on a river boat. He had been living the good life, fast and furiously as a young man. At the age of thirty-eight, Bhante became ill and was told he had six months to live. Bewildered by the hand that fate was dealing, he sought an alternative route to the one he was on. Bhante bid farewell to his family and traveled to Thailand. His saddened family thought he was going off to die—and indeed he did as well. But instead he found his way to Buddhism and joined a monastery.

"The monastery provided rigorous training, and Bhante studied hard. The Buddhist teachings completely changed his way of thinking and behaving. They served to greatly shift the course of his health and his life path. He then came to the realization that he had not been completely loving and found the resolve to make a miraculous change. Thirty years later he returned home for a visit to the great surprise of his family and friends. The reconnecting was deeply healing. Following this, he traveled to the United States and settled into life at the New York state monastery.

"Greg Lynn had been living in New Jersey, feeling his life needed a boost. He had been on a spiritual and healing path for quite some time and wanted to open up to new possibilities. One day as he sat in deep meditation, Greg Lynn said a prayer. He asked for a great teacher to come into his life who was a healer and a master of meditation. He punctuated this with the request that his new teacher be at least one hundred years old.

"The following week Greg Lynn's phone rang. He was invited to a luncheon in Princeton, New Jersey, where he met Bhante. The great teacher had reached the age of one hundred five months prior!

"When I met Bhante he was staying with Greg Lynn and the Peace Weavers in their unusual bungalow outside Lambertville, New Jersey, across the Delaware River from New Hope, Pennsylvania, where I spent my teen years. When Bhante celebrated his one-hundred-second birthday, he began experiencing some health challenges. He asked to come live at the New Jersey retreat for rest and healing. Currently many of the Peace Weavers live in upstate New York on an expansive tract of land covered with rolling hills, lush green grasses, and tall trees.

"Over the years, Bhante had become a very dear part of Greg Lynn's heart. He was a wise man and a gifted teacher of both meditation and healing—exactly what Greg Lynn had asked for in his meditative prayer. Bhante requested to come live with Greg Lynn and was brought to the wooded retreat in New Jersey. There the community took care of him and shared in the beauty of his wisdom and teachings.

"I had been hanging out on the skirt of the Peace Weavers for a long time, taking part in their meditation sessions and providing them with drumming for their celebrations. We had wild music and dance parties in the name of Peace at venues including Princeton University, Waldorf Schools, and parks. On sacred holidays that celebrate nature, including the equinoxes and solstices, we sat tightly packed in a Native American sweat lodge and stewed our bodies, minds, and spirits for peace on earth and purification. We ate vegetarian delights and gave each other energy healing and bodywork. Many of us were therapists and all of us were dancers and music lovers. Together we played with reckless abandon and reveled in the joy of being.

"I loved visiting the Peace Weavers' unusually beautiful house. It had three round, silo-like rooms that were connected by two long, rectangular-shaped passage ways. These halls had loft sleeping spaces peaked with windows on either side. I remember how their placement made the house look like the face of an owl with piercing eyes as I drove in from the main road at night. When I stayed over it felt like I was in a tree house cloaked in the quiet of the thick forest, connected to nature.

"The Weavers burned lots of sage, cooked delicious dishes, and drank herbal teas with all who came to visit and learn. They taught peace through all the senses. Each summer they would drive in a caravan across the country, stopping to teach peace through song and storytelling. The end of their yearly journey took them to Wyoming and the Dakotas, where they spent time with Lakota elders. These wise ones taught them the technique of passing a talking stick around a circle to encourage each individual to share from their heart and receive acknowledgement. I still use this technique when leading groups. Upon returning home from these sojourns, Greg Lynn would leave to go spend time with his beloved teacher at the monastery. After, he would return home to us with new stories and wisdom.

"One of the first things Bhante taught me is that thoughts, foods, and liquids are the fuels that run our lives and each is equally important. He said that too many people are more concerned about their cars than they are the vehicle of their body. He helped us all to be more conscious about what we were doing to our physical forms and, most importantly, in our minds. He taught us to look at our thoughts while sitting in peaceful meditation in a room flooded with green dichromatic light. This was one of his favorite techniques.

"He had figured this out when he was a young disciple sent out on a solo retreat into the woods. One evening he sat for meditation and found the light of his lantern too bright, disturbing his ability to concentrate. He placed his green silk scarf over the lantern to diffuse the light and create a more peaceful atmosphere for his meditation. The green light washed his body and filled his mind. Upon his return to the monastery, he shared his experience with his mentors. He was then dubbed 'The Monk of Green' and was given two focuses for his learning and ultimate mastery—mediation and healing. It was quite rare for monks in his order to have more than a single focus.

"Bhante discovered dichromatic colored light bulbs when he moved to the states. He insisted that they were the best for what he called his Green Meditations. It was the eighties and movies like *ET*, *Star Wars*, and *Close Encounters of the Third Kind* were popular. Walking into a Green Meditation at the Round House with Bhante felt like stepping into a spaceship in one of these films.

"His sessions were simple—just the art of sitting and being in the flood of green light. No fancy mantras or pretzel twisting yoga; just finding a comfortable position and sitting still. The guidance he gave was to empty the mind and breathe. News spread fast and people came from all over to partake in his meditation sessions. Though the focus was quiet contemplation, I recall noticing that some people seemed to always be in competition, trying hard to be good at the meditation. It amazed me how people would create so much struggle for themselves.

"After the quiet sitting portion of the meditation gatherings, we always had an opportunity to ask questions of Bhante. He would answer our queries with an outpouring of love and humor.

"One night Bhante asked us how we meditate on our own. An eager man brought up the fact that he liked to run. He went into a long discourse about how running was a big part of his existence and how it was his only way to meditate. He went on and on while Bhante listened very intently. After the man finished, Bhante took a moment before he responded. He looked around the room and talked about the peacefulness of simply sitting in meditation. The runner became frustrated. He began to argue with Bhante that this was the only meditation for him.

Bhante responded, "I do not understand this running. It seems to me, so many people are running."

I turned and looked at the runner and he was beaming, feeling acknowledged.

Bhante asked, "What is it that you are running from?"

"The man looked flustered; he did not know what to say. Bhante continued, 'I think you must be running from yourself!'

"The discussion went on for a while. The runner argued and Bhante chuckled. Eventually most of us came to understand the teaching. The man did have a point—running is indeed a way to get into a meditative zone—but Bhante called him on wanting to be praised for it and for neglecting the fact that just sitting still is very necessary.

"You see, meditation just happens. There is no prize like in a race. Bhante guided us to understand that floating in the state of being is the reward. That night I was very impressed with Bhante's teaching and resolved to spend more time around him in order to study his techniques and philosophy.

"Bhante stayed on, instructing us and holding public meditations regularly. Occasionally he would leave and travel back to the monastery in upstate New York. While there, Greg Lynn would go to visit and always return with more pearls of wisdom.

"Time passed and one day we got word that Bhante had become very ill with pneumonia and was in need of constant care. Greg Lynn went to him and Bhante asked to return to the round house for healing. Knowing that the colon is the child of the lungs in Oriental philosophy, the Round House crew bought a high tech colonic machine and several of them did a crash course training on it. Later they would offer this therapy to the community to clean us out.

"Bhante was brought back to New Jersey and after several weeks of therapy began to feel a lot better. The Round House troupe recruited many of the fringe gang, including me, to be Bhante-sitters during his convalescence. I gladly accepted. Just to be with him and watch him sleep was a great honor.

"I showed up for my first shift on a weekday afternoon. Willow was in the Round house to orient me to my duties. Bhante had a thorough cleansing with the new equipment that morning and there was little chance he would even need to leave his bed. She said the most I would have to do physically for him was to assist him if he experienced a coughing attack and to administer some herbal remedies. Easy enough, I thought. Willow was working as a personal companion to an elderly lady by day. She informed me that she had decided to bring the woman over later that afternoon to meet Bhante.

"That day was filled with calm stillness for me. In his presence I was truly able to be empty. My mind was completely void of thought. I was totally present and just breathing. The birds sang and the leaves danced in the forest. Bhante was so grateful for every little thing I offered to do for him. He had so much dignity even when coughing up sputum. I have never experienced such a gracious convalescent. As instructed, I gave him his medicine and he napped a bit. While he slept, I basked in his silent wisdom and listened to the sounds of nature outside. Just being in his presence was a meditation.

"A few hours passed and I was stirred from a contemplative state upon hearing Willow's voice coming from the kitchen. She called to me to come give her a hand. When I got to the cozy hearth I was introduced to the elderly woman that Willow cared for. She was adorable—petite and feisty.

"Willow scurried around the kitchen and prepared juice elixirs for all of us; then she asked me to help her introduce the woman to Bhante. I ran back to Bhante's room and began to get him propped up in his bed, ready to receive his visitor. Willow helped the little old lady shuffle into the bedroom. It seemed like an eternal ten feet of travel as the tiny woman padded through the doorway and over to the bed.

"After what seemed like an endless amount of time, it appeared that the woman was ready to ask Bhante a question. The buildup of slow-motion movements and shuffling created a great deal of anticipation. It was like a *B.C.* comic strip when a guy climbs the mountain to ask for the meaning of life from a meditating guru.

"The woman began to open her mouth and ask her question. Her hands emphasized the importance of what she wanted to know. I gasped in anticipation as the words were leaving her lips. Her question was, "So, tell me something...what's it all about?"

"I giggled. Bhante immediately got a smirk on his face. He lifted his hand and motioned for the lady to bring her ear closer to his lips. Willow grinned and the woman looked seriously into Bhante's eyes. Gently I lifted Bhante a little more as Willow supported her tiny ward a little lower.

"It seemed like another elongated moment as we got them into position. Finally the woman's ear was close to Bhante's mouth. With a Cheshire smile, Bhante proceeded to say, 'Every day, in every way, I'm getting better and better!'

"The lady found sudden strength. Perhaps the bee pollen Willow had mixed in her prune juice was kicking in. She snapped upright and looked puzzled. Loudly she exclaimed, 'What?' while waving her hands in the air.

"Bhante motioned for her to come closer. Once again, Willow and

I supported the two into a position where Bhante could speak into her ear. Once more, Bhante said, 'Every day, in every way, I'm getting better and better.'

"A puzzled and slightly disappointed look came across the woman's face. Again she exclaimed, 'What?' then, 'What's this?' as her hands gestured in the air again.

"Bhante's smile beamed brighter as once more he pronounced, 'Every day, in every way, I'm getting better and better.'

"I started laughing and Willow looked over at me. She started to crack up a little as well. Bhante repeated his simple sutra[10] one more time and nodded his head to the woman staring at him. With a puzzled look still on her face, she began to repeat the phrase 'Every day, in every way, I'm getting better and better.'

"Bhante became very excited and, seeing this, she repeated it again. 'Every day, in every way, I'm getting better and better.'

"Willow and I joined in.

"Soon we were all chanting the words over and over. The three of us danced around the room as Bhante swirled invisible patterns in the air gracefully with his ancient hands. We sang it out as we twirled and laughed. The phrase transformed into a sacred mantra. Golden light beamed in the room. The energy rose to a higher vibration. Time and space disappeared. We were in the void.

"I received a lesson in simplicity that day. The first time I had learned this was under the loving tutelage of Reverend Beth Gray, one of the first people to bring Reiki healing to the United States. She was a devout follower of the teachings of Louise Hay as well as a good friend of the author's. Her messages were always sweet and to the point. Her mantra had been, 'K.I.S.S.—keep it simple, sweetie.' Bhante was the second great teacher to give me this form of insight and thus enforced the primary lesson I had received on the subject.

"Bhante taught us that we are immortal beings and that love is eternal. In addition, he enforced that the vessel of the flesh is fleeting

---

10 **Sutra** सूत्र *sUtra* Thread formula, string, or discourse.

and we must care for our bodies at every level in every way possible. Our minds are powerful and the daily practice of maintaining positive, loving thoughts takes a great deal of focus. It is far more work than holding onto negative thought.

"Bhante lived to be one hundred ten years old. Those who had the grace to be in his presence were gifted. His beautiful energy is a valued essence that remains in the hearts of all whom he touched. I am very grateful for his simple yet poignant doctrine. It is a foundational cornerstone in the philosophy I now teach to my students and clients."

Love and Relationships

We are co-creative beings, and it is our birthright to utilize these skills. Art and expression is all about the process and not a final outcome. Think back to when you were a child. Perhaps you were given fingerpaints or clay. You did not stare at the medium and think, "I am not good enough to create a masterpiece," but rather dove in and experienced the colors and sensations. If youth is what you wish to rekindle, then partake in the creative outlets that you loved as a child. We must find a way to allow ourselves to plunge back into this imaginative part of ourselves, as it inspires a great deal of happiness.

It is a scientific fact that like attracts like. Therefore, we must act as if we wish to generate change. Over the years we have watched many people, including ourselves, transform our state of existence by altering our thoughts. The necessary energy needed to keep us on a steady positive path is the knowing that every thought is a seed which, potentially, can grow into a mighty tree. We must take care as to the types of seeds we allow to be nurtured and fertilized with our words. Once spoken about, these thoughts begin to be fed as they take root and sprout.

Therefore, it is important to be impeccable with our language and with our thoughts. Meditation is the tool we recommend to help gain control over the mind and our thoughts. When we are able to realize that the world around us is a reflection of who and how we are, it is easier to take steps of transformation. To unfold what appears as a hidden secret we must realize that everything we perceive to be outside ourselves is actually also very much a part of every microcosmic aspect of whom and what we are. This is true at the energetic level as well as the physical world around us.

Our ideas about relationships and what we project to the outer world are ultimately what we end up manifesting. When we become discouraged we bury ourselves in a distorted cave, believing that we are not worthy.

Ambika explored many aspects of the human experience of relationships and the powerful energies of attraction in her book *Lilith*. A conversation between characters discussing relationships explains,

"'They seem to be like towers that we build, only to knock them down. Then we build another on the rubble of the aftermath.'

"'Yes, you human beings often opt to scramble from one relationship to the next. It is as if you are moving holes.'

"'Moving holes?'

"'Yes, moving holes. If you dig a hole, you have a pile of dirt. So you dig another hole to put the dirt into, but then you have another pile of dirt.'

"'I get it—we humans can search and crave and devour, but unless we desire to merge, we stay hungry. So, therefore, if we build up the ideas of relationships and tear them down when they appear not to be what we want, we are left with the rubble of destruction. The demolition leaves the ground more conceptual and, like insects, we humans yearn to reestablish and rebuild.'

"'It is the animal mind that drives you to try again.'"

Hormones and chemistry are radically affected when we feel loving, loved, and acknowledged. The experience of love brings the potential to awaken from the dream that the material world and our relationship to it is what we truly are.

Love has the magic ability to bring us instantly into the present moment. On the wings of love we are able to fly beyond attachments and the unnecessary cravings that cause us to believe that we are not good enough or that we are not deserving of happiness. The chemistry of love changes the sense of belonging for all living things. Though it is seemingly intangible, when we tune into love, we are able to find a place of acceptance.

All beings experience craving and are drawn into wanting to make connections. We all hold a deep and sacred prayer that love and happiness will find their way onto our path and stay in our lives. Our feelings, needs, and desires come from a deep, base level. We have animalistic instincts that churn and drive us. Inside each of us is a passionate desire that draws us to want a feeling of belonging in relationships. This is natural and essential for all living things.

In order to make radical shifts in our present relationships, we must dive into the dirtiest, ugliest part of ourselves and rediscover our own inner beauty. When trying to manifest anything, including a job, a partner, or a place to live, we must ask ourselves, "What am I bringing to the table?" It is important to remember that all relationships are to the self. In order to really comprehend this, we must understand what it means to remain in a state of feeling and being.

All we really want is to feel acknowledged and heard. So, in order to place our newfound awareness into action, the first thing we must practice is active listening. If we are aggravated or agitated, we must forgive ourselves. When we want to feel appreciated, we must have gratitude for everyone and everything; when we crave love, we must give love.

We need to train the mind to stay positive. There are scientifically measurable algorithms regarding positivity. It takes more muscles to smile than it does to frown, and more muscles are needed to wave than to exhibit a rude hand gesture. When we have a negative thought, the clock begins to tick and we must turn it around within the next ninety-one seconds to create a positive spiral. To make this happen, we can opt to press our fingers into the corners of our mouths and force a grin while repeating, "Happy, happy, happy," for the required minute and a half. This will surely send you and everyone around you into peals of laughter. Once the feelings shift to positive, you have created the necessary change.

Thoughts travel in a helical pattern. A negative thought spirals and generates more negative thoughts in sixty seconds. A positive thought needs ninety-one seconds to regenerate. It takes a lot more work to be joyful and generate happiness.

One of the best and most healing ways to give unconditional love is through hugging. If love is what you crave, then love is what you must give. When you hug, do it with the intention of sharing your heart. Imagine the unconditional love circulating through your hands and flowing from your heart. While in the embrace, let yourself smile. This all helps to train the body, mind, and spirit to synchronize in a state of unconditional love.

There have been many hugging saints and healers who know the power of healing love contained in a hug. It is important for us to be sure we give plenty of these on a daily basis. Look around you—there is definitely someone who could use a hug! Each time you share your love unconditionally, it comes back to you a hundredfold. This is pure blissful happiness.

The Preoccupation with Decision Making

We learn at a very early age to be choosy. As children we began to express ourselves through the ideas of "I like it, I don't like it," and this in turn became the way we viewed the world. This process of choosing and making choices is a product of our learning system and developed into a perceived survival necessity. It is, however, an illusion. This concept was not a part of us when we landed in these bodies.

As babies we did not stop to think, "Should I ask to be fed or cleaned or placed gently to rest?" We simply felt the need and followed the instinct.

The animal kingdom is driven by instinct. A tiger does not scheme and plan ahead. He does not think, "I will store up five deer so I will have more for later." The tiger hunts when he is hungry and stops eating when he is satiated. He rests when he feels contented and complete. There is no struggling—only instinctive action. This is how we are when we are children. We cry when we are cold and we seek warmth. We eat, poop, and sleep, and are joyful when we are playing. In the first few years of life this comes easily and naturally to us.

The Original State of Being

As babies, when we are warm and fed, clean, and feeling safe and secure, happiness is the true state. With our initial breathing cycle we begin to roll along with the rhythmicity of nature. We have no need for external things to create a sense of happiness, and our bodies function in a seemingly automatic fashion.

As we begin to develop, it is through observation that we learn about ourselves and the world around us. Our ability to feel happiness can be blocked by various external causes. This takes away from a knowing of what we are really made of beyond the realm of the physical world.

Much of what hangs us up in life is triggered by the idea that we need to make the right choices. We wonder and spend a lot of energy trying to make decisions in all aspects of life. These involve everything from what to wear and how to look to who are the right people to spend time with, what schools to attend, which jobs to pursue, and where to live.

This excess of decision-making creates a great deal of stress. This stress keeps many from having the ability to rest properly, digest with ease, and in turn plants seeds of disease. Once the cycle turns to imbalance, the individual finds even more stress by having to choose new health regimes and, ultimately, doctors and treatments to counterbalance all of this inequity.

By this point it is very difficult to know what to do. The cycle quickens and becomes even more confusing. We get caught in a tumultuous storm of even more choices, and this in turn tangles us in even more stress.

The solution that seems to be cloaked in secrecy is to stop making decisions. Though this sounds simple, once the mind begins to wrap around the concept and we use intuition rather than logic, we no longer feel overwhelmed and desperate. How can we find our way back to

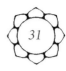

simply tuning into the sensations of what feels right? If you stop to think about it, this is exactly how we behaved as tiny babies.

The key to being able to function in a pure state of trusting intuition and allowing the body to be led in the right direction has nothing to do with the mind. It is the mind that got us into any portion of this mess in the first place. Sure, the mind is good for calculating and storing information, but when it comes to a decision, it is best to ask the body and even better yet to ask the heart to lead.

Realizing Happiness
Ambika shares a personal realization

"I had been feeling boxed in—like I did not have any space. This is a place I can find myself when I am pressing too hard or listening to what others think. I begin to feel pulled into the depth of darkness by the undertow of negative thought when I begin to believe I should follow what others tell me to do, instead of riding the conscious waves of inner guidance.

"The symptoms are just as easy to read as to deny when they crop up. Clothes and books pile up in my bedroom and receipts waiting to be itemized and entered into spreadsheets begin to form a mountain on my desk. My body begins to feel tired and listless. I hear negative chatter inside my head but can't seem to do anything about it. Sleep is interrupted, digestion needs a little help from herbs, and my morning meditations are short and fitful. This is when I realize that something has got to give.

"If I let this continue into an even more chronic state, my diet may shift into less healthy choices and I become lazy about exercise. The projects that were making me smile and sing and dance around the house don't call to me to come and play, but rather taunt me for losing my creative drive. So how the heck do I get myself out of this tailspin? Indeed, it can be a challenge to pull out of a downward spiral. After all, it is not always easy to change the directional travel of a ton of emotions.

"When I was younger, I would brood. I was so good at it that I could have turned it into a profession. It had become a chronic pattern that in turn created a fertile ground for all sorts of disease and disorders. I did not realize until many years later that this was learned by watching the adults in my life. Adding to my cutting-edge ability to be miserable, I had also learned that this actually got me more material things. As I look back, I am not angry or disappointed, nor do I feel let down by my family. I am actually quite grateful.

"Now that I am able to step back from this and witness the patterns, I can see that this is familial and not at all a trait that I developed on my own. It is also apparent to me that I brought this with me into this body, and this life path as it is necessary for me to have these experiences. But, before I came to this realization, I once asked a great teacher of mine how to get past all of this.

"'How do I get to the place where I am completely free of all of this mind chatter and nonsense?' I asked quite sincerely. 'What is the path to get clearly past this and find the place of complete quiet and peace?'

"I really thought at the time that this was a great question, so I was not at all ready for what came next. My teacher listened intently, and then he laughed. It wasn't just a chuckle; it was a full out belly shaking laugh. I was sitting in a room full of people and really hoped that my question would get me a solution. Back then I was hoping there was a formula I could follow, a necessary prescription, and that all the meditating and other yoga practices of diet and exercise I had been doing were somehow a solution that would produce a perfect, permanent outcome.

"While my teacher continued to laugh at my question with tears streaming down his cheeks, the people around me began to giggle nervously. I shrunk with complete humiliation. That was a very long moment. Finally he stopped, took a soft inhalation, looked at me, and asked, 'What is the point in that?'

"'To get past the mind, to find peace,' I answered, hoping to regain my footing.

"He laughed harder. I shrank more. I felt like an idiot. I was trapped, sitting near the front of the crowd, and there was no escaping.

Between my self-loathing, humiliation, and fear I wondered, 'What am I not getting?'

"Then he gave it to me—the true wisdom. 'This is a part of being human,' he said. 'It is a gift to feel and have reactions. This is how we know we are human.'

"That was when it truly clicked for me. All feelings are part of our nature. It was like a thousand cards being dealt on a table in rapid-fire succession. Each face held a scene and situations. Some were solved and resolved, others still pending.

"I melted out of existence and didn't really hear the rest of the discourse that day. What I had needed was in the words, 'This is how we know we are human.'

"The great teachings of the world have similar suggestions to help us get in touch with our true nature and accept it. As I look back at my youth, I can see this was offered to me by the schools I grew up attending. We always had time set aside mid-morning for a hiatus in our daily schedule from classrooms and learning. We would gather for a warm cup of tea and chat in the fresh air under the large, spreading oak trees, or just sit quietly enjoying a break from our minds and work, just being with nature.

This was followed by a community service job. There were many chores, including sweeping steps, raking leaves from a path, placing library books back on shelves, or helping the cooks in the kitchen prepare for lunch. The jobs rotated, and everyone had worked in a variety of positions by the time they had graduated.

"I thought back to the ashram where I had lived and studied and how we had been on a rigorous schedule of meditation, chanting, learning, and service to the community. Back then I was so consumed by the actions of study and service that I had little time to get caught up in my own stuff. This is an absolutely brilliant side effect of living in this form of conscious community.

"So here I was faced with my own true nature. It is said that in every great rehabilitative process we must first identify the problem.

Okay, so I was seeing this—something had to give. This is what makes us so different from the world of nature around us.

"Animals function from a different part of the brain than we humans do. On my daily morning walks, I love to tune into the environment and remind myself what it really means to be connected to nature. I watch the bunnies awaken in the morning and go about their bunny ways of chomping succulent plants and enjoying the sunshine glinting through the leaves at the edge of the wooded areas they call home. Bees flit from flower to flower, drawing in sweet nectar, which they drink with happiness, and lizards cling in gravity-defying postures from leaves and lampposts before leaping and scurrying into cracks and crevices. These creatures are in a constant state of being. They are not caught in ego-minds.

"Now when I hit an emotional bump or slam into an uncreative wall, the first thing I have to do is notice the reactions. This is what my teacher was trying to get across to me—that the reactions are what make us human. It is one thing to realize this, but then where do you go with it?

"The trick is to not get caught in a cycle of re-reaction. This is the spiral that drags us under. Think of it this way—a wild cat gets up in the morning, cleans himself, and when he is hungry, goes out to hunt. He catches a meal and eats until he is full.

"The big cat doesn't think, 'Oh, I look fat today; maybe I should find a low-cal antelope.' He just cleans his fur, hunts, eats, eliminates, and rests. If only it were this easy for us humans. The squirrels don't get into a big bargaining match over who has the best nuts or which tree they should rent to keep their storage supply safe; they just gather, store, and crunch.

"Centipedes cross the sidewalk when they feel like it and birds sing when inspired. All of nature moves and survives in happy harmony without regret or overthinking. It is only when we domesticate an animal that it can potentially become depressed. So how do we get back to our true nature with so many stressors and pressures from the society that we have created?

"What I do for this closed-in feeling is to spend a day cleaning. I get down on my knees and scrub the floors with a brush, and then go over it again with a steamer until it is gleaming. I work and sweat for a few hours and when it is all dry, I feel happy. The act of cleaning consumes me. I lose the train of chatter and the sparkling tiles make me feel that I have infinite space.

"I don't just stop there. I give to others. I make donations or offer to take on a task for a friend. The act of reaching out and helping someone in need creates an immense amount of space for me. I have been known to clean the public spaces I use when I am out and about, picking up trash and wiping down the counters in public restrooms. This gives me the opportunity to remember that we are all connected and is a humbling act of gratitude. When I am making others happy, I smile. That makes them happier and, in turn, I eternally grow even happier!

"Chaos is a necessary shakeup of the order of things. The confusion and frustration we sometimes feel is a cycle of life; there is nothing wrong with it. What we must do to get back on track is to first realize it is there, and then give it space to be for a moment. Then we can roll up our sleeves and get down to the task of cleaning up our own ego-based projections. This reconnects us to the collective.

"When I get past my own uncomfortable waves of emotions, I am able to truly realize happiness. This is when things just begin to flow. The phone rings with a new client, old friends pop back into my life, and I drift into a song and dance around my house. The happiness doesn't come from accumulation; it comes from stepping out of the mind and out of my own way. It comes from stillness and a soothing quiet when for no reason, I just stop and close my eyes and listen to the breath."

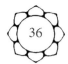

SPROUTING
The ability to grow or develop

Although happiness is our true nature, it can be cultivated and developed through the maintenance of optimum health and the prevention of diseases. The sister sciences of Yoga, Ayurveda, and Jyotish[11] come from the timeless knowledge of the Vedas[12] and provide us with a wealth of information. Together, these great teachings give us many guidelines to remain healthy and happy throughout life.

Ayurveda, the science of life, possesses ancient wisdom that gives us integral tools to live life to the fullest potential. The teachings of this science explain ways to remain happy and healthy within the external world through suggestions of lifestyle and nutrition. Yoga guides us to quiet the mind and teaches us to detach in such a way that we realize we are not our thoughts through the practice of meditation. Jyotish illuminates our path and helps us to understand who we are, what we came here to be, and our gifts to share with the world.

According to World Health Organization, health is a total integration of the physical, mental, emotional, social, and spiritual parts of our existence. The tools of Ayurveda gift us with an array of choices to assist in dismantling everything that is in our way to achieve perfect health and

11 **Jyotish** ज्योतिस् *jyotish* Light as brightness and as the divine principle of life and source of intelligence. The science and movement of the heavenly bodies. Astrology.
12 **Vedas** वेदाः *vedaH* True or sacred knowledge. Texts originating in ancient India. The oldest scriptures of Hinduism.

be in total harmony with the external environment. An understanding of Ayurveda places us on a path to maintain health.

Understanding the principles of Ayurveda and her sister sciences help us comprehend that we are more than our physical body. In any given moment, the physical body is the end result of all experiences metabolized in the past. If we want to know what kind of experiences have been digested by an individual, we can look at their body today. To know how their physical body will look and feel in the future, we can observe their experiences being processed today.

Truly, we have the power to change our physical body by bringing in different experiences through our senses of sight, sound, taste, smell, and touch. The way we process these experiences and our emotions—through the use of our mental faculties—does the rest. The physical body is always changing—each time we are presented with new inputs and let go of the old metabolized parts.

We replace ninety-eight percent of all the atoms in our body once a year. The stomach lining changes every five days, a new skin covers us every thirty days. In six weeks we have a completely new liver and every six months we have regenerated a new heart, kidneys, and lungs. Why then do they maintain the same patterns and disease states? To understand this, we must realize we are not just our physical body.

Thoughts are powerful and determine our destiny. Our thoughts, emotions, memories, belief systems, and stories that have developed around those belief systems are interwoven into our physiology. The way we experience all sensory inputs from the external environment depends upon our memories of similar previous experiences. The method our body uses to digest this information is dependent upon our emotions and belief systems.

We learn about ourselves as a result of what we are taught with regard to who we are, and are influenced by sensory experiences from the external environment. Our concepts, ideas, belief systems, likes, and dislikes are constructed during childhood and shaped by our family and society. This creates a sense of self which governs the way we experience life as well as our self-perception. These inputs may not be fully correct for maintaining our unique and individual bodies. Our belief system creates boundaries that limit our ability to allow certain experiences in relation to others. This in turn creates a conflict between what we need as opposed to what we bring into our bodies. These clashes can be the seeds for triggering an illness or a state of happiness at a later date.

In addition, there exists a "higher self" within what we perceive as who we are. The higher self is full of unlimited possibilities. It is a permanent part of our existence, but is hidden and seemingly silent. The "false self" is the ego. It is loud and limited by belief systems that prevent our ability to experience the full potential of our being.

The state of health is then achieved by being established in a state of higher self. This is the same state we are trying to reach to be happy, joyous, content, and blissful. This higher state is reached through the practice of meditation. It is a part of the consciousness-based approach to health, joy, vitality, love, and strength in our lives.

The true self exists beyond the physical body and mind. It is the authentic choice-maker and thought-maker, and it exists beyond the false ego-self. When we are able to access this part of our higher self through awareness, we create coherence and spontaneity in all of our actions. This in turn allows appropriate inputs into the body that generate true health and wellness. This is the first governing principle of Ayurveda and its potential gift for our day to day living. The concept of individualized medicine is the hallmark of Ayurveda and the second governing principle.

Elemental Energies

The elemental energies are the first manifestations of primordial energy transforming into the realm of matter and are responsible for the entirety of creation. They make up the whole universe, including galaxies, stars, planets, water, rocks, soil, plants, animals, and everything we human beings are made of. Ayurveda states that "whatever is in the macrocosm is in the microcosm." Therefore, whatever the stars are made of comprise the same five elemental energies that we are made of.

The elements are divided into five groupings and occur in a particular order. Each evolves from the previous. Space is unique in that it never changes or breaks down, and therefore is the primary element created from primordial energy. The remaining four elements are generated from space and possess the qualities of the elements that come before it. The five elemental energies are:

Space The experience and vision of space is given the name *Akasha* in Ayurveda works and is derived from the Vedic model of cosmology. It is the open expanse in which everything is contained. It is not void but rather full of information and energy. All communications take place in space. Space is eternal and can never decompose. The etheric quality of Space is present in the remaining four elements.

Air is motion and is named *Vayu*. It is the carrier of everything vital, from ideas to nutrients, and has the ability to move and animate. Air is the subtle life energy and though we cannot see it, we can feel it move us. Touch and Air are inseparable.

Fire is transformation and is named *Agni*. Fire represents light, heat, and luster. It is present as the radiant energy from the sun, and is heat and light. It is an essential and powerful converter and has the capacity to burn. Fire is the power of transformation, understanding, and metabolism.

Water is transportation and is named *Jala*. It joins and nourishes all of nature through its interconnecting ability. Water is cooling and brings moisture. It is a stabilizer and gives flow and smoothness as it softens everything it comes in contact with.

Earth is structure and is named *Prithvi*. It manifests as solidity, mass, and form, and gives support, food, and shelter to all creatures. Earth is present in rigidity and stability and gives structure where it exists.

From primordial energy, space is formed first. Movement is created in space to produce air. Friction to the movement of air creates fire. Fire liquefies into water, and earth is created by the solidification of water.

The five elemental energies are organized into three biological humors. We all have these, and they control our physiology. The amount of each humor present determines our unique constitution. The constitution, in turn, is responsible for the psycho-physical character of an individual. By determining constitution through the knowledge of the elements and humors, Ayurveda makes recommendations of life style and foods. An individual's physicality, personality, and habits give many clues to their constitutional makeup, just as an expert astrologer can see the potentials in the natal chart of an individual. The most proven method used in Ayurveda to determine this is the examination of pulse.

The body has three broad functions—motion, energy production, and structure. If you were to ask Vijay, when he was practicing as a Western-trained physician, what makes the heart tick twenty-four hours a day, seven days a week, he would have answered that it is the autonomic nervous system.

The motion functions of the body include the breath moving in and out, nerve impulses, circulation of the blood, the distribution of nutrients to cells and tissues, and the removal of waste products. The body also has energy functions that include the metabolic processes and the enzymes that digest food and extract energy from it. Each cell has energy-producing chemical reactions, and the solid physical structure of the bones, muscles, fat, and flesh mobilize the body.

These all have characteristics identical to the functions of the three Doshas[13]. Vata[14] is expressed in all motion and is the principle of movement. Pitta[15] manifests in metabolism, digestion, energy, and heat production. It is the principle of transformation. Kapha[16] gives solidity, structure and balance to the body and humors. It is the principle of cohesion.

Ayurveda teaches that what exists in the macrocosm is also present in the microcosm. We see this correlation in the natural world around us. In the earth's ecosystem, Vata is expressed in the motion of the wind and in water currents. Pitta is present as sunshine and fire. Kapha brings the

---

13 **Dosha** दोष *doSha* A body humor.
14 **Vata** वात *vAta* The humor of air and space.
15 **Pitta** पित्त *pitta* The humor of fire and water.
16 **Kapha** कफ *kapha* The humor of earth and water.

solid structure of the earth, rocks, and water.

These humors can go out of balance in nature. A hurricane is an imbalance of Vata; blazing heat is an excess of Pitta; a flood or blizzard is an inequality of Kapha. The same occurs in the balance of our bodies. These imbalances formulate the core beliefs and explanation of disease in Ayurveda.

Ayurveda therefore gives us information and suggests steps we can take in order to normalize the Doshas that are out of balance. This addresses not only the symptoms but the root causes of disease, which in turn creates lasting improvement.

Concept of individual Constitution

The three Doshas are present in each of us. The unique proportion of each determines our individual constitution. A person whose mind-body constitution shows a preponderance of the air principle or Vata will likely possess attributes that resemble the wind. Others, who have a dominance of the fire principle or Pitta, have an impassioned nature that manifests in both the body and mind. Those with abundance of the earth principle or Kapha are typically grounded and steady, remaining unruffled by change. Understanding our unique nature provides us with the information we need to make conscious choices to create optimal health and well-being.

Please Visit Appendix I to learn what your Dosha is.

Modulating Sensory Experiences

The third governing principle of Ayurveda provides us with tools to modulate, modify, or transform the sensory experiences according to our individual constitution. When utilized, these bring us to a harmonious balance of body and mind. In addition, it teaches us how to reconnect to our higher selves. Through this wealth of scientific knowledge we discover how to stay in accord with the laws of nature, moving and flowing with her rhythmicity. Fine-tuning our behaviors by applying the tools of

Ayurveda gives us the opportunity to live life to its fullest potential. One of the most important sensory inputs is taste.

Transformation through Taste

Ayurveda places a great deal of emphasis on nutrition, digestion, and metabolism, teaching that they are accomplished through the sense of taste. The principles that govern digestion and nutrition are

Food is equal to medicine. Most of the imbalances in the body can be corrected by simple adjustments to the intake of food and spices. "Let food be thy medicine," is an age-old Ayurvedic dictum.

Like increases like and opposites decrease one another. A truth of Ayurveda is that when a food has a certain quality that increases a particular humor in a constitution, then food with the opposite quality will decrease that humor.

Agni is a major principle in Ayurveda; it is the digestive fire. Digestive fire is needed to digest anything we bring into our body. If the Agni is high, even a suboptimal intake can be fully digested, absorbed and assimilated in the body to create energy. However, if the Agni is low, then even the best quality foods do not provide the right nutritive value as the food is neither properly digested nor properly assimilated.

Think of a fireplace in which the fire is burning strong. You can place a wet log on the fire and it will convert it into heat and ashes. However, if the fire is of low intensity, then even a dry log will just smolder and not produce heat or ashes. In the same way, if our Agni is low, then the foods we eat cannot be properly digested, processed, or assimilated into the tissues. Conversely, too much fire can burn the food and char the digestion. The strength of appetite reflects the underlying state of our digestive fire.

The Six Tastes

Nature has packaged all possible food sources into six tastes. Before the discovery of proteins, carbohydrates, fats, minerals, vitamins, and trace elements, Ayurveda taught that we need all six tastes present to make a balanced meal. The six tastes are sweet, sour, salty, pungent, bitter and astringent.

Please visit Appendix II for examples of foods and spices categorized into the six tastes.

Here is something you can try:

Make Khichri, which includes all six tastes. **Visit Appendix III** for a delicious recipe. Enjoy this Tridoshic dish. Notice how it nurtures your senses and soothes your feelings. Try eating it, made fresh, for several consecutive days and watch your digestion relax and harmonize.

How to Eat

Ayurveda teaches that in addition to balancing the six tastes in each meal, it is also important to eat in a particular way in order to aid proper digestion. How to eat is more important than what to eat in many circumstances.

It is recommended to eat in a settled environment, away from the disturbances of television, computers, cellphones, and other visual distractions. This leads to better digestion and assimilation of nutrients. We all know how upset our stomach feels when we are troubled or eating in a rush. It is common sense to eat only when we are hungry. Think of a car's tank that is full of gasoline. What will happen if you put more gasoline in that tank? It will overflow. The same is true of the body. If we eat when we are full, the extra nutrition will remain undigested. This overtaxes the system, which in turn makes it difficult to digest. The undigested food is converted into toxins that deposit in our tissues, creating obesity and other diseases. This is one of the main life style issues in the Western cultures.

When a meal is placed in front of us, it is important to give thanks. Take a moment to imagine how many people and hands it took to get all of the ingredients to your kitchen and table. Thank the earth, sun, and rain for nurturing the food, and the animals that took part in pollination and fertilization of the plants. Infuse your meal with love and gratitude prior to taking your first bite. It is a proven fact that food and drink are more nourishing and easier to assimilate when a prayer is offered prior to consumption.

The Simple Magic of Hot Water and Awareness

Sipping hot water during a meal helps to maintain our digestive fire. When obesity or poor digestion are a challenge, try sipping hot water when you think you are hungry. If the body is indeed ready for food, the hunger remains. When thirst is the trigger signal, then the warm water satisfies the urge. Eating with awareness will apprise us of the subtle messages our body gives us while we are eating to let us know whether the foods we are consuming are appropriate for us.

Here is something you can try:

Sip hot water while you are eating and see how light you feel during and after the meal. This will be especially important if you have overeaten or eaten the wrong foods. It may even prevent heartburn or gas and bloating. Dr. Jain has had several overweight clients who got rid of twenty to thirty pounds in six weeks by simple modifications and eating only when they are hungry.

In our culture, obesity is a problem because of lowered metabolism and eating beyond what is needed. By listening to the intelligence of the body, we can change our habits and eat only when we are hungry. Identifying what is true hunger requires tuning in to the natural rhythms of the body. When the fire element is strongest in the environment, our hunger is at its highest. Eating the biggest meal at lunchtime helps satisfy us biologically and is great for assimilation and digestion.

Nutritional Guidelines

In addition to the importance of the six tastes and our tips on how to eat, there are also certain nutritional guidelines that emphasize the importance of what not to eat. Ayurveda sees that digestive difficulties are the beginning of many other health problems and believes that by managing our diet we can greatly improve our health and vitality. It is important to eat fresh, home-cooked meals. Home cooking puts life, energy, and love into the food and creates a meal that is nourishing to the body and the spirit. Fruits should be eaten separately to avoid digestive issues as enzymes needed to process the simple sugars in fruit are different than the enzymes needed to process complex carbohydrates, proteins, and fats. It is important to avoid leftovers. Storing, freezing, and microwaving food destroys its ability to nourish the body and leaves you feeling unsatisfied after a meal. Avoid too many frozen items, especially at night when the digestive fire is lowest. Fermented foods also tax our digestion and create incompatibility with other foods. Refined sugar, sweetened, prepared foods, and snacks possess little to no energy and hinder digestion.

Timing is Everything

There are optimum times for meals. Breakfast is best between 6:00 and 10:00 am. At this time the body is in a cleansing cycle, so take foods which assist in elimination like fresh fruits, juices and herbal tea. When you feel excessively hungry, enjoy whole grain hot cereal.

Lunch is best when the sun is high in the sky, between 10:00 am and 2:00 pm. This is the optimum time to digest a full meal of grains, beans, and vegetables.

The evening meal should take place before sunset. The digestive strength at this point in the day can be weaker or irregular, so it is recommended that dinner be lighter than lunch. After 6:00 pm, the digestive fire begins to quiet down for the night, so it is suggested to eat earlier rather than late.

Remember—what to eat, how to eat, and what not to eat as well as what are good combinations is the shift in paradigm Ayurveda brings to our understanding of nutrition. Different tastes bring varied emotional states and possible transformation. Ayurveda goes further and states that different foods can create the production of different brain chemicals to create those conditions. Think about how chocolate in small amounts can create a state of ecstasy and happiness, while larger portions can create restlessness, hot flashes, and bitterness.

Understanding the Cosmic Dance

The fourth governing principle of Ayurveda is the synchronization of our internal environment with the external environment.

Health is a harmonious relationship of mind, body, and spirit with our extended body, and our connection to the environment. It is also a harmony of all the rhythms in our physiology. Just as rhythms influence the physiology of the universe, they in turn affect the physiology of our body. We have stated, "As is the macrocosm, so is the microcosm." The rhythms of nature, her music, and dance are all reflected within our physical body. When our internal rhythms are in synchrony with those of the environment we experience well-being.

Every cell, organ, and system in the body operates according to predictable rhythms, with periods of dynamic activity and times of quietness. These same patterns of rest and activity can be found within the cycles of nature. The sun rises, shines brightly, and sets. The seasons flow one into another and the tides rise and fall in response to the moon's orbital pull.

The fires of digestion increase and decrease, influenced by the mind and the physical system. Our hormones—specifically secretion of cortisol, growth hormone, thyroid stimulating hormone, and prolactin—fluctuate according to a twenty-four-hour rhythm cycle. Our moods, mental agility, and motor skills move through relatively predictable highs and lows throughout the day and over the course of each month on various biorhythmic cycles.

Diseases tend to occur at certain times of the day or in a particular season. For example, incidences of heart failure tend to increase in the morning hours when platelet aggregation has been observed to increase. Allergies tend to occur in certain seasons. A tooth is more likely to begin aching between 3:00 am and 8:00 am and least likely to begin aching between 3:00 pm and 4:00 pm. A dose of corticosteroids will control asthma and improve peak expiratory flow significantly more if injected at 8:00 am and 3:00 pm rather than 3:00 am and 8:00 pm.

In our modern society, many of us are unaware of the natural rhythms of our body and are guided instead by habit and convenience. We tend to ignore internal signals for external ones. The result is compromised health, fatigue, and the accumulation of toxins in the mind and body.

Ayurveda considers attunement of the individual's lifestyle to natural biorhythms a crucial element of disease prevention and treatment. In addition to the internal biorhythms of heartbeat and respiration, there are four primary celestial rhythms that take place in accordance with distinct patterns within the human body. Adjusting our daily routines and tuning into nature's rhythms can bring us harmony.

Circadian Rhythms are circular and cyclical. The twenty-four-hour cycle of night and day is created by the earth spinning on its axis. These inspire us to sleep and wake, as well as setting the cadence for many bodily functions.

Lunar Rhythms take place in a 29.53059 day cycle caused by the moon's continuous revolution around the earth and occur in thirteen lunar cycles throughout the year time. Modern cultures have implemented a twelve-month calendar to measure this mathematically. The monthly lunation and bi-yearly eclipse cycles affect all life on our beautiful planet, inwardly and outwardly.

Tidal Rhythms are governed by the location and phase of the moon with respect to its elliptical orbital path. The waters of the earth and our physical and our emotional bodies are influenced by the gravitational fluctuations of the lunar orb's proximity and placement.

Seasonal Rhythms are created by the proximity and tilt of the earth's orbital path around the sun. When tilted closer to the Sun, we experience warmer seasons and when further away, cooler.

Planetary Rhythms are tracked by the graceful dance of the celestial orbs in our solar system. Each planet affects us in a unique way at all levels of body, mind, and spirit. The unique transits of these planets are measurable and comparable to where they were at the moment of birth. This gives vital information with regards to potentials and propensities.

Adopting a regular daily and seasonal routine helps us to be in synchrony with our environment and creates greater energy, happiness, and well-being. Early signs of disease are reflected by the disruption of biological rhythms at the mind-body level. When there is disharmony or disturbance of these rhythms in nature, it leads to imbalance in the body with signs of fatigue, lack of sleep, and poor digestion. When we are in harmony with the rhythms and cycles of the seasons and hours in the day, we are happy.

Daily Cycles and the Doshas

One way to view these cycles is through the dynamic interaction of the three principles of life, which are Vata, Pitta, and Kapha. These can be thought of as motion, transformation, and structure, respectively. Each of these Doshas represents a bundle of qualities that describe a style of action or functioning. For example, Vata is said to be light, cold, dry, rough, moving, pervading, clear, and subtle. Any time we experience something that can be described by one or more of these qualities, then Vata is said to be at work, influencing and governing.

Ayurveda states that during the course of a day, the principles of motion, transformation, and structure increase and decrease in an orderly and repetitive way. This means that at a certain time of day, we would expect the physiology to express certain qualities more than others, thus promoting certain functions or processes.

Different needs of the physiology of the body are more or less active at certain times of the day. At noon, the quality of heat is livelier than its opposite, cold. Heat is involved in digestion, metabolism, and all forms of energy transformations. Given that heat is more active at noon and that it is the basis of digestion is the reason digestion is strongest at that time.

Ayurveda advises that life is easier, smoother, and more fulfilling when we acknowledge, honor, and make use of the biorhythms and cycles of nature. There is a purpose to the changing qualities of the day, month, and year that affects health. An important understanding of Ayurveda teaches that it is not enough to do the right thing; one has to do the right thing at the right time. This makes sense from the angle of limited resources. The energy from food can be used to digest, to breathe, to work, and to play, but if we work and eat simultaneously energy resources will be diverted to the work and away from digestion, causing digestion to suffer.

Recall that Vata and Kapha are cold while Pitta is hot. Vata and Pitta are light and Kapha is heavy. Vata and Pitta are mobile while Kapha is static. Vata is dry while Pitta and Kapha are oily and liquid. As the heat of Pitta reverses the cold of Kapha, other qualities increase and decrease in turn with the passing of time. Therefore, what we see is a pattern that permits a quality in the environment to build, then release or reduce. Nature provides for this as a way of restoring the balance of quality and action. It purifies itself in an ongoing, cyclical way. The same ebb and flow is perpetually taking place, providing for harmonization deep within the microcosm of the body and in the macrocosm of nature and the universe.

Going with the Flow

We are familiar with the cycle of change associated with the rotation of the earth on its axis that creates day and night. This is an important progression to tune in to because the rising and setting of the sun, in large measure, dictates various qualities that predominate at different times of the day. Rest takes place at night and activity during the day. The revolution of the earth around the sun causes seasonal variations of daylight periods—for example, longer days during the summer and longer nights during the winter. Thus, in the context of seasonal variations of day and night hours, we should experience and honor the tendency of the body-mind to want to go to bed earlier and even to sleep longer during the winter season. This expresses the dynamic interaction of the environment with the body-mind.

The body reflects what is happening in all of nature because it is always connected to nature. What dictates to the body and takes us away from our ability to tune in is the sway of society. This in turn influences our behavior and takes command over the timing of activities.

Therefore, it is important that the mind always be aware of the body's needs so that the body-mind can function effortlessly by not being compelled to do things excessively or at the wrong time. The concepts of changing the clocks, as in the case of Daylight Saving Time and time zones, are unnatural because they direct our attention away from the internal signals of nature to the external fiction of an hour. In this way we force our bodies to ignore natural tendencies in favor of economic considerations.

The daily sequence of Vata, Pitta, and Kapha moves with nature's cycles. As we become more aware of the quality of the Doshas and relax, allowing ourselves to ride these circadian rhythms, a natural happiness overtakes us. The time periods of the three Doshas happen twice daily, with one in the daytime and one at night. Vata time is between 2:00 and 6:00 both a.m. and p.m. Kapha time is between 6:00 and 10:00 a.m. and p.m. Pitta is between 10:00 and 2:00 a.m. and p.m.

During the early morning Vata hours, nature is alert yet quiet. This is the best time to experience profound meditations. Vata is responsible for elimination, movement, locomotion, speech, enthusiasm, creativity, breathing, and functioning of the nervous system. This is the natural time to eliminate waste that has been removed from the tissues and accumulated in the bladder or colon during the night. It is important to void the bowels and bladder first thing each morning for this reason.

Vata has the qualities of lightness and motion. It is an essential ingredient for achievement in life. When we get up during the early hours of the morning, the body is alert, rested, clear, light, and energetic. This sets the tone for the entire day and gives way to effortless and productive activities. Many people report that their creativity and mental clarity are especially lively during these early morning hours. Ayurveda supports the aphorism, "Early to bed and early to rise makes a man healthy, wealthy, and wise." We can add "happy" to this as well.

Recent research has confirmed that the Vata period is more connected with mental activity than physical work. Mind-body coordination and dexterity is greatest around 4:00 p.m., which is midway through the afternoon Vata phase. The Russians have discovered that muscle strength is weakest during this Vata period in the afternoon.

Pitta functions control digestion, metabolism, transformation, intellect, courage, enthusiasm, skin, tissue colors, and vision. At noon digestive capacity is greatest; therefore, the noon meal should be the largest. We noted that the afternoon period is best suited for mental activity, and we can see how nature provides for this by calling for the main meal at this time which, when digested, nourishes discriminative and creative mental effort. It is interesting to note that many cases of high blood pressure are attributed to skipping the noon meal. The habit of eating a large evening meal forces Pitta to become active during a time when the body wants to slow down. This degrades the quality of both digestion and sleep.

On the other hand, the evening Pitta period is more about house cleaning than digestion. Research shows that liver activity and small intestine activity increase around 1:00 a.m. to 3:00 a.m. Many people report that mental clarity increases after 10:00 p.m. This is natural because Pitta governs the intellect. However, forcing the body-mind to be dynamic at this time compromises its internal cleansing efforts. This in turn increases Ama,[17] which in stress and toxins that accumulate if this function is disturbed.

Kapha governs structure, fluid balance, secretions, binding, growth, potency, patience, heaviness, compassion, and understanding. Its qualities are heavy, dull, and slow. The evening period of Kapha is largely suited to sleep. Research confirms that if sleep starts in the hour or two after sunset, then rest will be improved. This is likely due to sleep being deeper and longer lasting. Rest helps rebuild, restore, and cleanse the body, so it makes sense that we should honor this aspect of our biorhythm by getting to bed early—before 10:00 p.m. Ayurvedic

---

17. **Ama** आम *Ama* Undigested, uncooked.

practitioners often report that getting a person to go to bed before 10:00 p.m. can cure chronic insomnia.

The habit of "sleeping in" may be viewed as digging a hole from which a person has to climb out each morning before they can become really effective. Therefore, the morning Kapha time is the best for dynamic activity. Movement during these hours helps to balance the body's tendency to be slow, heavy, and dull. After the body-mind has rested, it is better able to perform and exercise, which is especially useful for eliminating toxins or Ama during this time period. This in turn produces lightness and helps to build a capacity for work, thus promoting balance.

Ayurveda gives suggestions for a daily routine based on this information accordingly. Awakening without an external alarm clock is possible when we become in synchrony with our internal clock.

Here is something you can try:

Try going to bed at 10:00 p.m. and awakening without a clock for one week. Write an entry in your journal each morning upon awakening and in the evening before retiring. Notice the difference this makes in how you feel.

Seasonal Rhythm and Lifestyle

According to Ayurveda, seasonal rhythms have important influences on our biological cycles. Each season expresses characteristics of a specific Dosha. Autumn and early winter is Vata time with cold, dry, and windy weather. The hot, moist summer expresses the qualities of Pitta, while the cold and wet weather of late winter and spring are expressions of Kapha in the environment.

The body needs to adjust to the outside environment. The food we take in is one way to help the body accommodate to the changes in seasons. Each season brings about nurturing qualities, and it is the natural tendency of the body to want to plug into nature for its rejuvenation. In the absence of this, the body tends to compromise its natural defenses, which are essential for the strength and well-being of the system. Another way to achieve balance is through lifestyle modification and preventative measures.

In order to explain transition points, we are using approximate markers of the seasons in the northern hemisphere. Changes occur due to shifts in temperature and weather. During the hot summer months in areas where distinct seasonal changes occur, June through September is a Pitta season. During this time individuals are prone to skin ailments like sunburn, acne, and rashes. It is recommended that cool, light fruits and salads be consumed to calm and correct the imbalances caused by excessive Pitta.

During autumn and early winter—September through December—is the Vata season. This is a time during which people are prone to symptoms of arthritis and rheumatism. It is recommended that individuals eat warm, oily, and hearty meals like beans and whole grains to lubricate the system and keep it hydrated, helping to counter the dryness of the Vata season.

When the Vata Dosha predominates there is an increase in the dry, rough, and cool qualities of our external and internal environments. Excess dryness can be disturbing to various tissues and organs. Most noticeably we can experience dry skin and lips. An internal drying can also be occurring, particularly in the colon or large intestine where Vata is prone to first accumulate. Though we all notice the seasonal effects of autumn, people whose constitutions are Vata-predominant and the elderly, who are in the Vata stage of life, are most susceptible to this change.

Daily activities have a profound effect on our health and happiness. A routine, practiced regularly, is stronger medicine than an occasional remedy. Consistency is of particular importance as we enter into Vata season. When the cool fall weather arrives and the holiday season is upon us, it can sometimes be difficult to maintain a peaceful, grounded state of being. Having a routine to follow restores balance throughout the day and safeguards us against the anxiety and stress associated with increased Vata.

According to Ayurveda, Abhyanga, or oil massage, is an essential component to a daily routine. This practice nourishes and strengthens the body, encourages regular sleep patterns, stimulates internal organs, enhances blood circulation, and can significantly reduce Vata.

During spring, which is the Kapha season, people are prone to bronchial ailments and common colds. To help pacify the Kapha, Ayurveda recommends foods that gently warm the body—like honey, millet, and greens—be included in the diet. As we move into winter, from December through March in the Northern Hemisphere, a season in which Kapha predominates strongly, all the Doshas must work together to preserve health. Kapha is the endurance which enables us to move through this season, but it needs the Vata qualities of light and movement and the initiative power of Pitta to do so. Without this we are likely to simply crawl into our dens and sleep away until spring!

When the weather warms in the springtime, March through May in the Northern Hemisphere, the Pitta liquefies the accumulated Kapha, which is then eliminated from the body. As a result, people are more prone to colds, nasal allergies, coughs, sinusitis, and other respiratory congestion syndromes. These are all signs of Kapha aggravation.

For these reasons, a good routine for spring involves steps to reduce Kapha. A Kapha-pacifying diet includes bitter, spicy, and astringent taste groups. These all help to reduce the qualities of Kapha. For a Kapha constitution, it is extremely important to use the pacifying procedures. In addition, one should drink only warm fluids. Warm sunshine and exercise also help to reduce Kapha.

Among the strongest health measures when the season of spring comes is Panchakarma,[18] an Ayurvedic rejuvenation therapy. Ayurveda regards Panchakarma as the best method of removing backlogged imbalances and impurities during this time of the year.

Abhyanga, the Daily Oil Massage

Massaging your body with oil is an important aspect of the daily routine that provides a stabilizing influence all year long. Massage

18 **Panchakarma** पञ्चकर्म *pañchakarma* Literally, five actions.

nourishes the tissues, stimulates the skin to release health-promoting chemicals, improves the circulation, increases alertness, facilitates detoxification, and improves immunity.

The classical texts of Ayurveda indicate that daily massage rejuvenates the skin and promotes youthfulness. The purpose of the Ayurvedic daily massage as part of the regular routine is to prevent the accumulation of physiological imbalances and to lubricate and promote flexibility of the muscles, tissues, and joints. For details on the procedure of Self-Abhyanga, please refer to Appendix IV.

By honoring the Ayurvedic notion of biorhythms and how qualities and functions increase or decrease in a regular, rhythmical manner, we support and facilitate proper physiology. In addition, by understanding the nature of the ongoing changes in the body-mind, we can select activities that promote balance when done at the proper times of day.

Here is something you can try:

Use organic, unfiltered Sesame Oil and give yourself a daily Abhyanga massage for a week. Notice the changes in your skin and the way you feel. We are sure you will continue to do this daily!

Rhythms and Cosmic Coincidences

We have always had a fascination with the cosmos. Our curiosity led us to develop systems to understand our connection with this vast realm. The ancient astronomers of long ago were astrologers. They were sought after to unravel the mysteries of existence and to help explain who we are and why we are here. These cosmic scientists read the intricate patterns constructed by the great orbs and interpret the beautiful music composed by their travels within the matrix of fixed stars.

Jyotish, the Vedic science of light, is Astrology and is the third sister of Yoga and Ayurveda. Throughout history astrologers have been interpreting the subtle causal effects of the movement of the planets. Through their calculations and observations, they help us to actualize and give comforting acknowledgement through the weaving of epic stories that guide us to understand our dharma[19], who we are, what we came to learn, and our gifts to share with the world.

Why should we stop at the elevation of the moon as influence on our earth and our bodies? The mapping of a natal chart was performed throughout ancient times and still is available to determine the propensity of health, career, and relationships.

A skilled astrologer utilizes scientific data along with honed intuitive skills in the reading of the physiology, psychology, and spiritual potentials of an individual. Through the telling of rich stories and by giving loving guidance, these seers are able to provide us with information and help us to understand our purpose.

Expert astrologers prescribe specific healing sounds through mantras that are determined through information held in an individual's birth chart mapping. Patterns and trends are identified and provide guideposts and explanations to unravel the questions of why and when in timeline fashion. The birth-chart mapping profoundly explains our personal psychology, physiology, and spiritual path.

Ambika shares thoughts of witnessing her astrology clients' transformation over the years.

"Astrology is the original psychology of the spirit. It can feel like magic when a client suddenly finds happiness either though acceptance of a current situation or in making a bold move suggested by what I see in their astrological mapping. The Dosha propensities and curative suggestions help us to find harmony and are easily read in a natal chart."

We are able to see and feel our connection to the cosmos through our emotional tidal patterns as we observe the monthly lunar phases. This is a good place to begin.

Lunar Rhythm

The Lunar rhythm is marked by the monthly cycle of the moon

---

19 **Dharma** धर्म *dharma* Nature, manner, those behaviors considered necessary for the maintenance of the natural order of things.

revolving around the earth. The time of a new moon escalates Vata, and the phase of the full moon increases Kapha. Tuning into the external rhythm of the moon helps us to balance our internal humors and leads us to a state of happiness.

Women know the feelings and the effects of the waxing and waning moon. This is easily observed in their cleansing and fertility cycles. It is scientifically proven that the moon phases correspond to an increase and decrease in female hormones. Male hormones are also affected, though it is less noticeable for most men. Tuning in on a regular basis, looking up at the sky, and connecting with the phases of the moon helps us integrate on a day to day basis. The gravitational influence of the moon on the waters of the earth changes the tides, including oceans, lakes, and rivers. When the tide is high, it is Vata time. This affects the waters of the body and the emotions as well.

The natural cycles spiral and vibrate cosmic coincidences that become obvious once we are able to tune into them. Location and timing are easily charted, helping to give us explanation and comfort as well as guidance. We use a road map to get from point A to point B. Therefore it makes sense to consult the cosmic information to assist us in understanding and reaching our highest potential and embrace who we came to be.

Above all, we must always remember that the natural environment is our extended body and that our bodies are a part of her. Nature has already provided everything we need in the perfect place and at the appropriate time in order to sustain us. The more we are in tune with natural internal and external rhythms, the more we can accept and metabolize the nourishment that is so readily available to us.

Panchakarma, or Cellular Detoxification, Is the Fifth Governing Principle of Ayurveda

The Ayurveda cellular detoxification practice is called Panchakarma. It is a fivefold technique that helps in maintaining health by preventing disease through the purging of endogenous and exogenous toxins from the body. Panchakarma also helps in eliminating emotional toxins that

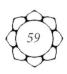
accumulate in our physiology.

Ayurveda teaches that routine detoxification can be precious for maintaining good health during seasonal changes. Getting to the root cause of illness is another benefit of Panchakarma that helps in the management of most lifestyle related chronic diseases. These include autoimmune diseases like Crohn's, ulcerative colitis, rheumatoid arthritis, chronic heart disease, diabetes, obesity, and chronic digestive disorders. All of these conditions can be improved with Panchakarma. When we change our lifestyle and adjust our food choices according to our constitution, we easily find a better state of health and happiness. The harmonizing effects increase when we synchronize with biological and nature's rhythms and practice detoxification on a regular basis. The addition of a meditation practice helps us to stay established in our true nature. This augments lasting effects and increases our sense of joy, bliss, and happiness.

Is Health Equal to Happiness?

Is it true that if I am unhealthy I cannot be happy? The answer is no. Having a disease does not mean you must be unhappy. It is through acceptance, giving space, and surrender that we can come to accept a condition and continue forward in a true state of happiness.

To dive into this idea we would like to share with you our feelings about what the state of health is. Health is not the absence of disease; health is when we are established in the higher self. This is where we become an observer of life. Therefore, everyone has the ability and potential to be happy.

If you had visited Dr. Jain twenty years ago when he was practicing strictly Western-style medicine and asked whether you were healthy, he would have examined you and done a battery of tests. He then would have declared that you were healthy if the results came back negative for any possible diseases. Now he explains that "A true state of health is when immunity is stronger than bacteria, viruses, fungi, and carcinogens. An example is that you are in a state of being healthy when you do not contract the flu if exposed to ten people who have it."

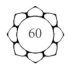

It is important to remember that a disease does not mean that you cannot be happy. We believe that the easiest way to experience this is through the practice of meditation. The mind-clearing effects of meditation help us to realize our true state of being and in turn remove the perceptions and misconceptions of what is important.

GROWTH UPWARD AND INWARD
Techniques to Unfold Happiness.

The Attitude of Gratitude

Gratitude is pure awareness of the Divine energy that surrounds us. It is an intermediate place between prayer and praise. When our attitude turns to gratitude, it shifts awareness from the contractive states of moping, selfishness, and jealousy to the expansive place of grace, joy, absolute bliss, and happiness. This in turn leads us into a state of compassion and pure detached awareness.

Discipline and the practice of unattached awareness are important to achieve gratitude. Most people find it a challenge to fully realize that we have the ability within ourselves to co-create our lives along with the universe. Many doctrines teach us to accept what we are given. This can become confusing and fool us into thinking that it is not appropriate to dream of anything more than what we appear to have.

The powerful primordial force of creativity is held in each and every particle and cell. Cosmic co-creation is our birthright. We must come to realize that our hopes and dreams and individual creative powers are an integral part of true beingness. They exist in a state of potential, awaiting activation. These energies are the budding seeds of light and love that directly transmit information and in turn guide us to utilize our gifts for the purpose of following dharma, our true path.

When we really want something to shift in our lives or have a strong desire to manifest an object or situation, it is easy to become confused. It is only through steady contemplation that we can identify and initiate deliberate action. We must learn to focus upon our awareness in single pointed observation and self-examination. This is the method by which our world begins to materialize and form. Once we develop the will to act according to our convictions, we must then find the energy required to produce the results envisioned. This requires control over sense organs.

At any point in the process, manifestation can become perplexing. The methods used to follow through can get lost in translation beginning with our initial desire and then moving toward the final outcome. Obstacles and feelings of shame and doubt confuse us into perceiving that asking for what we want is pleading and begging. It is true that when we live continually seeking the gratification of all our sensual demands our passions can ultimately consume us. We then become slaves to our senses. The ability to regulate our indulgences without denying them keeps them from causing suppression and frustration. Therefore, we must learn to enjoy the world without letting it obscure our clear vision.

The truth is that manifesting what we want in life is no different than walking into a store and asking a salesperson for a specific item. We are not ashamed of this—why then should we feel embarrassed to ask for what our heart desires?

Imagine you want to purchase a red sweater. You go to a store that has sweaters and walk right up to the salesperson and say, "I would like a red sweater, please." The sales person scurries off and comes back with an assortment of sweaters for you to look at and try on. You have great ease in fanning through them and vetoing the ones you do not want. Perhaps there are V-necks, and you are looking for a crewneck. Maybe there are cherry-red sweaters made of sheep's wool and what you really want is closer to the color maroon and made from alpaca. As you go through the various choices with the sales person your description and communication becomes clearer as you hone in on exactly what you are looking for.

Perhaps you are wearing a green crewneck sweater that has been a longtime favorite. When you let go of the idea that you must find exactly the same sweater in red, your idea dials into focus. This is an integral point of realizing that you are not trying to duplicate a past experience. As you partake in the shopping process, you experience the present moment. When the image is locked in, the very next sweater you come to is exactly what you are after. You smile and take it happily to the checkout counter.

Once we have a crystal-clear vision of what we want, we easily step into the silent realm where all possibilities exist. It is very important to find the quiet space between our thoughts in order to do this. There are many methods that can be used to come to this stillness, which is the place we let our desires be known.

From this quiet place, we can easily announce our intentions to the pure energy field of potential where creation takes place. When we imagine the finest details and every angle, including scent, color, and how it feels to have what we want, we are able to receive the exact design of our dreams.

Similar to dropping a pebble into a pond, the ripples created by our thoughts travel quickly from this place of tranquility, echoing out into the world to align and orchestrate all the necessary details to bring our desires into manifestation. Before leaving this wonderful space to come back to the world, it is important to release any attachment to the outcome and express gratitude. By doing this daily, we focus our thoughts and our energy while regularly mingling with the essence that makes it possible to build the life of our dreams.

When we experience a positive manifestation, it is necessary to have an attitude of gratitude. This is something everyone must learn to express. On a surface level, it is plain courtesy and good manners to be thankful in return for someone's help. When we look deeper than the norms of society, we find that the attitude of gratitude is needed for self-realization and personal growth. Through the act of giving thanks one realizes that there are things greater than one's self. It is also helpful to have the synergetic energy of many people to help with accomplishment.

For example, in most cases, a novel only has one author. When we turn to the acknowledgments page, however, we see the author's gratitude and how the writing and publication process was the combined efforts of many more people.

The humble nature that springs from the attitude of gratitude is of particular interest. When one truly recognizes the greater forces at work around them, one realizes how insignificant they are. This in turn makes one humble toward life and the world. Therefore, the attitude of gratitude is not just necessary for good manners, but for self-realization as well.

The threat of losing something creates a stronger sense of gratitude. Philanthropy and giving freely to others helps to counter the act of satisfying our personal desires with excessive collecting and spending. Happiness is to know how to celebrate. Happiness is prosperity.

There is no need to avoid unhappiness; that leads to a hunger and desire for happiness. We all have the capacity to be happy. We have a right to be happy. We have an obligation to be happy, and we must remember that happiness is a choice.

Happiness is a state of being where everything is all right. We must learn to enjoy the happiness of pursuit rather than pursuit of happiness. It is not our genes but our beliefs that control our lives. We must ask ourselves if we can let go of all that we are holding on to. Is it possible to become a nobody in order to become a somebody? If others are always responsible for my problems, then I have a serious problem of allowing others to create problems for me.

"Nothing" is very important to me for it is from there that I have started my journey. What I see is not what is. I see the world and expect it to be not as it is. It can be that knowing too much stops us from knowing more. Do I know so much that I stop learning further?

There are many places in the world where people live in what we would consider complete poverty, yet they are exceedingly happy. What do they know that we don't? They don't have a way to find happiness outside of themselves. They realize that it is within them with both a deep knowing and an unknowing. This creates a trust and, in turn, a great deal of happiness. Happiness comes when we accept where we are at any stage of life. No more "ifs" or "buts" or "could be" or "would be." This acceptance brings us closer to happiness.

It is also important to find happiness while dying. The *Tibetan Book of the Dead* has a wealth of good information regarding procedures to focus the mind on particular images and thoughts while experiencing the last moments of life and our final breaths.

The act of selfless service, also known as *seva*[20] or Karma yoga[21], is a practice that inspires a great deal of happiness. It teaches us that the act of serving is to say to oneself, "you are my exercise on myself and I am yours on yourself." Seva is the act of giving selflessly. This provides more satisfaction and happiness than only placing our energy in material gains. We must remember that donation can be ego-driven and that seva is a true way to give life energy. This brings forth more contentment than anything else. The easiest way to stay true to this is through the daily practice of meditation, which helps us to find this peaceful place effortlessly and quickly. Meditation helps us to identify what happiness feels like.

It is always advised to be modest and humble. This is the key to selfless service. We must approach it without ego analysis and while maintaining childlike trust. This means that it is important to function from a place of instinct and intuition. This is the act of tuning in.

---

20 **Seva** सेवा *sevA* Service.
21 **Karma Yoga** In English *Seva* is often referred to as Karma Yoga. This is the combination of the words: **Karma** कर्म *karma* which means action and **Yoga** योग *yoga,* a physical, mental and spiritual discipline originating in ancient India.

BRANCHING
Synchronicity and Sharing

Manifesting happiness can be difficult when a person is suffering from a chronic illness. During such times, control can be gained through the practice of meditation. This helps in determining the root cause of a given illness. Once realized, implementation of change becomes easier.

To exemplify this point, we share our own stories of what brought us to Ayurveda.

Vijay shares a Personal Story About the Path that Led Him to Ayurveda

"As I sat watching the movie *Doctor*, I thought that someone had made a movie about my life. In the film, William Hurt plays a surgeon who incurs a chronic illness, forcing him to quit his practice. Just as the character portrayed by Hurt in the movie, I too was at the pinnacle of my career. In 1989 I was chief of medical staff and a surgeon in a hospital in the greater Cincinnati area. The title came with many responsibilities, including the chairmanship of various committees.

"I had just taken on a partner in my practice of general surgery, and it was booming. In addition I had a lifestyle that matched my position with late meetings, late dinners, and many parties. I saw myself as being able to walk on water and believed that I could accomplish anything. I was living the American dream.

"That was all shattered as I sat in the waiting room of the Mayo Clinic in Minneapolis, Minnesota. I was hoping to get clarity regarding two months of difficulty swallowing and an upper respiratory infection. All my tests were normal and several visits to a local ear, nose, and throat specialist and a gastroenterologist—a specialist who handles matters of digestion—had failed to make a cohesive diagnosis.

"Intuitively, I knew that there was something grossly wrong, but didn't know what it could be. The impersonal nature of the ordeal started to take a toll on me as I was hurled from one laboratory to another. I realized for the first time in my life what it felt like to be a patient. I was frustrated, scared, and restless.

"The only test that showed abnormalities was my elevated level of creatinine phosphokinase (CK), which is a muscle enzyme. I was probed and X-rayed from head to toe; a biopsy was taken from a muscle in my arm. Finally the dreaded moment came when the neurologist informed me of his opinion about my diagnosis.

"'You have an auto-immune disease called polymyositis,'" said the attending physician.

"There is no known cause of polymyositis. The immune system starts destroying muscle cells, which in turn causes them to become inflamed. Because of the nature of the inflammation and muscle damage, I was advised to stop my surgical practice until the muscles healed to prevent further damage to the tissue.

"My ability to swallow was affected due to the weakness of the muscles in the neck. The more central muscles of the upper and lower extremities were also involved, contributing to my infirmity. In addition, walking was not allowed as it was believed it would cause further damage. Treatment essentially consisted of steroids and anti-inflammatory drugs like methotrexate. I was ordered into a wheelchair to prevent further damage to the muscles even though I could walk. This put me into a state of shock, disbelief, and denial. For the first time in my life I felt I had no control over the situation or my emotions. Tears welled up immediately. I couldn't speak for what seemed like a long time. When I did finally communicate, I argued with the neurologist, saying, 'I am very important person at my hospital and can't take off without giving them a sufficient amount of notice. Who is going to do everything I do?'

"The neurologist's reply will always resonate with me as the most philosophical advice I have ever received from any one. He replied, 'You will see that you are not very important. Two weeks after you stop your practice, people will forget who you are. Take care of your health. This is the most important possession you can have.'

"I began the medical protocol but my clinical condition and laboratory tests didn't improve for a long time. My inner voice kept telling me that I needed to do more for myself as the treatment was only addressing the symptoms. I knew at an intuitive and a philosophical level that if the cause of the disease was not known, then the cause was within me, and the answer or the healing of the cause was also within me.

"I tried visualization and imagery techniques, physical therapy, and mind-body practices. I attended Louise Hay's course on positive affirmations. These were not helping; I was not getting better. I felt that I need to get to the root cause of the problem. It took eight more years before I found a system that changed my life forever.

"I returned to part-time surgical practice after six months only to have a relapse in another six. I received high doses of steroids daily and weekly administration of chemotherapy which had tremendous side effects. Sometimes these were worse than the disease itself. I was already weak with the malady, and the steroids increased that weakness.

"In addition, there was insomnia. I was unable to sleep for days at a time. I gained a significant amount of weight. I had elevated blood glucose levels and my blood pressure climbed. The once-a-week intravenous chemotherapy caused severe nausea and fogginess in the head. There was a risk of toxic effects on the heart and lungs if taken in large, accumulative doses. During this time I experienced depression and anger.

"I went through seven more exacerbations of the disease and seven more courses of steroids and chemotherapy. Every episode started with weakness and difficulty in swallowing, and then the blood tests would show elevated CK enzyme levels. With each cycle there was a six-month remission, only to have the symptoms recur in another six months' time.

"Life had become difficult at best. I started to feel lonely. It is not a common disease and after research and the help of the Arthritis Foundation, I was able to locate twenty-five patients with the disease in the greater Cincinnati area. With compassion, I started a support group for fellow sufferers of polymyositis.

"My surgical practice was slowly dwindling and I was increasingly depressed. No one was giving me any answers except to take the medicines when there was a relapse of the symptoms. It was way too dangerous to continue taking the high doses of steroids continuously.

"No physician—neither my neurologist nor rheumatologist—ever discussed with me what I could do to prevent the exacerbations. No one talked to me about the role of lifestyle or nutrition on my disease process. I was frustrated, not knowing the answers. Being ingrained in the Western medical approach all my life, I was not even open to alternative or complementary approaches to health and wellness. When the opportunity appeared to investigate such a possibility, I rejected it as it was not evidence-based medicine.

"In modern medicine, there is no known cause of polymyositis. Therefore, all that can be done is to suppress the symptoms using high-powered toxic chemicals and then wait for the body to heal on its own. I had, however, not changed my lifestyle and still worked long hours, competing to climb the ladder of success in my career. I continued to keep late nights and attended parties. I consumed alcohol and lived a materialistic life. Even though I achieved success as defined by society, accumulated material possessions, and became chief of surgery and chief of medical staff at my hospital, there was no inner peace.

"Finally, I started searching for alternative approaches to healing. I was tired of suppressing the symptoms. It was like putting a lid on a pressure cooker, which would control the steam only for a short time. In turn this leads to a release of steam with more vigor once the pressure rebuilds. Something had to change.

"I was then introduced to Ayurveda, a system of mind-body

medicine, which addresses the tangible as well as intangible parts of our existence. Initially I was skeptical. Once I opened up my mind, I was able to grasp that health does not mean only physical well-being of an individual. It was becoming apparent that the state of homeostasis is where emotional, spiritual, and social wellness is in sync with the physical. I also learned that being a part of nature means that one has to live in accordance with the rhythms and laws of nature.

"Today I believe that all disease comes with a message encoded in it from the soul that lets you know you are on the wrong path. Once the message is received and you begin to change your lifestyle to fulfill the purpose of your life dharma, disease can be asked to leave.

"What I learned is that our thoughts, emotions, and belief systems are intertwined into our physiology.

"If we want to change our physical and mental state, we need to bring different experiences into our life. Just as Rita Mae Brown wrote, 'Doing the same things over and over and expecting different results is the definition of insanity.'

"I made significant changes in my lifestyle, including a shift to a mostly vegetarian diet. I began to follow daily and seasonal routines. The changes included a winding down of my surgical practice so that I had more time to study and apply mind-body principles to my life. I also began a daily meditation practice, which was one of the single best things I have ever done for myself. This is when my life began to change significantly.

"The principles of Ayurveda teach that eating honors the life force and fuels one's body with vitally energized foods that support our physiology. I began to understand that honoring my constitution involved bringing in only the right amount of food and information from the environment to support and balance my body. It was at this time I was introduced to the powerful science of detoxification. After undergoing several detoxification courses of Panchakarma, my symptoms began to fade and my disease went into remission. Though I had continued taking the Western medicines I had been prescribed, I was able to wean off them slowly until I no longer needed them.

"The disease went into complete remission and I was able to stop all medications. It had taken almost three years for this to occur. I went back to full time surgery in 2001 and practiced for eleven more years. Ayurveda changed me and my perceptions about life, health, and disease. This, in turn, completely changed the way I approach patients and their unique situations."

Ambika Shares a Personal Story About Being Led to Ayurveda

"I felt like jumping off a bridge. My body was covered in itchy splotches, each the size of the tip of my pinky. I had just left the office of a nutritionist who was an outside-the-box thinker. He meditated to figure out solutions for patients and hand-made many of the remedies he dispensed. I had a lot of hope when I first went to see him, but on this day I left feeling completely depressed. It seemed that in the beginning he believed he could help me. But after the first two months passed, I hit a wall and just wasn't seeing any changes. This was not unlike so many other modalities I had tried in the past.

"For eighteen years, I had taught holistic health at the college level in three different states. As I look back, I am sure it is my knowledge and intuition that kept me alive and helped a great deal, though I never seemed to be able to get the right balance. My digestion had always been a challenge and I couldn't remember having three consecutive days when I felt vibrant and full of energy. But on the day when the doctor looked with sadness into my eyes and said 'I'm sorry, I just don't think I can help you,' I felt my heart sink.

"So there I was, sitting at a traffic light on top of a bridge going over Route 101 in Scottsdale, Arizona, and the thought of getting out of my car and jumping off actually seemed like a choice. Thank goodness I changed my mind as the light turned green.

"More doctors and more years went by. I managed to stay out of the hospital except for one scare a couple years later that had me in an emergency room for a few hours, unable to urinate. As I look back, there were so many oddities I had endured. I am sure it sounded crazy to the parade of practitioners I visited.

"The recurring themes always included poor digestion; lethargy; chronic ear, nose, and throat issues; and a general feeling of malaise. Less frequent occurrences were skin outbreaks, hair falling out, and debilitating back spasms. I continued to see a naturopath and received B-12 shots and chelation drips to have enough energy to work as a musician. It seemed I went from doctor appointments to gigs and back to the doctor.

"Over the next few years, I found myself traveling back and forth to Florida more and more to visit my mother. I realized that while I was in the humidity and less extreme heat of Florida, I felt better. I decided to pick up and move across country.

"Immediately, I began to feel some relief. I could breathe, and my skin seemed to give more space to my insides. But I still struggled with digestion and the feeling that things were crawling both inside and on the surface of this body. Back then, I really had no idea what feeling good actually felt like. So on the better days I was grateful, and on the challenging days I persevered.

"Somehow I managed to continue to survive. For the previous two decades I had seen almost every type of practitioner imaginable, from conventional to alternative. I was scanned energetically and chemically. Many of these tests pointed to similar findings—poor pH giving host to parasites; poor digestion—I already knew this, believe me—and various diseases namable and unknown. Some said I had so many types of parasites they could not identify all of them. Others said, "It's like Lyme disease," and "Maybe you have herpes."

"I tracked down an infectious disease specialist known to have cured hundreds of dirt-eating children of numerous viruses and organisms while volunteering in third world countries. He sent me for blood work which he believed gave conclusive evidence that I indeed had Lyme disease, mononucleosis, Epstein-Barr virus, pneumonia, and a type of herpes zoster. He looked me in the eyes on my follow up visit and asked, 'How did you get here?

"'I walked in. You saw me,' I responded.

"'No! How did you get here?' he asked again.

"'I got in my car and drove across the state. Then I parked in your parking lot and came into your waiting room and checked in...'

"'No, how did you get here?' he asked again.

"I was baffled, not at all understanding what this guy wanted me to say. 'I drove,' I offered once again.

"'Why? What are you trying to get me to say?'

"He looked back at the papers in his hands containing the data from my blood tests.

"'Well, it is quite obvious I got here on my own!' I repeated. I had driven four hours and most certainly had walked from my car into his consultation room.

"'People like you don't walk,' he said. 'They are carried in here!'

"I was glad I was sitting down. That was not at all what I was expecting, and certainly not at all what I had hoped for.

"'What do you mean?' I asked.

"'People with results like this are...'

"Thank goodness his words ended then. I don't want to know what he was thinking. His solution was to put me on antibiotics for life and some other chemical that seemed it would do final damage to my immune system. I let him know I would think about it and begged for some strong parasite tablets he had used to cure a group of kids in Africa. He reluctantly wrote the prescription and made me promise to call for another appointment in two weeks. I agreed and thanked him for the prescription.

"Thank goodness the next person I met was Dr. Jain!

"On my first visit, I felt so broken. I had driven a long way to the Yoga institute where he had begun to offer consultations and week-long detoxifications. I began to go into my very long, detailed health history as I handed him my blood work. He looked at it and handed it back with an assuring smile.

"'Do you think I have all of these diseases?' I asked.

"He told me no, he doubted it, and explained that impurities in the body can build up and often throw off blood work. I wanted to believe him, but after all I had been through I was finding it a challenge.

"Dr. Jain felt my Ayurvedic pulses in each wrist and checked my tongue. He seemed most concerned about my sadness. This, he felt, was the first thing I needed to focus on changing. That really penetrated right to my core. We talked about modifications to my diet. He said that I needed a few months to let these changes begin to take effect before I would be strong enough to partake in my first Panchakarma. He explained that this would be a retreat geared at internal cleansing of the body for cellular detoxification.

"After our initial consultation, Dr. Jain walked me over to the dining area where we would have our lunch. He held up a little jar of tawny colored powdered herbs and introduced me to a blend called Hingvastak.

"'Mix a half of a teaspoon of this in some warm water and drink it before you eat,' he instructed me. 'It will help your digestive fire and build up your Agni,' he smiled.

"I did as he instructed and took the first sip. The pungently flavored liquid made its way down my throat and into my stomach. There was a gentle heat so soothing and pleasant I found myself squeezing my eyes shut. I began to cry as I had never felt this sort of warming feeling from food. It tasted like the best broth I had ever experienced—peppery and tangy. But it was the sensation that shot me over the moon. I felt warm all over. I felt loved, and this in turn gave me an overwhelming sense of happiness. It was the first major step in my healing.

"Within three days of returning home I began to feel different. The burden of malaise that had become the norm for me began to disappear. I continued using the Hingvastak herbal blend. Food began to actually feel good in my belly when I ate and my digestion grew stronger and better.

"Over the next six months I used various herbs at different times of the day and evening. I was taught to take some in the morning on an empty stomach, others before meals, and one blend after meals. I was no stranger to odd-tasting and sometimes brackish blends as I had been self-treating for years, utilizing various tinctures and teas. But nothing ever before had produced such profound sensations. Each time I used the simple plant-based blends of the Ayurveda herbal empire, I could feel something and would have an instant understanding. It was as if the cells of this body were enlivening and changing for the better, and I could actually feel it. But even beyond feeling it, I had a deep-felt sense of knowing.

"Six months later I took part in my first Panchakarma with Dr. Jain. Now, four years later, I have completed my fifth. Each year I feel progressively better and better in every way. I have become more and more productive and a lot happier. My diet has naturally shifted over this time, without force, to vegan. Rather than thinking about when and what I should be eating, I find myself knowing what would feel good and choose these foods. It is easy to sense when I am really hungry and only eat at these times. All choices are made intuitively, with nourishment as well as cleansing.

"I had always hoped to one day find a more balanced state of health and to know what this would feel like. It is my hope that you too will also find this magic in your exploration of Ayurveda."

BUDDING
Manifestation and Living in the Material World

The wise monks of Tibet teach us that there are four steps in the process of manifestation. They say that first we must identify what we really want. Then we must really, really want it. The third step is to completely let it go and the fourth step is the appearance of what we asked for.

This simple method sounds easy enough but any step along the way can easily confuse us. That which we desire is indeed what we draw to ourselves. It is also true that what we fear is magnetically attracted into our lives as well. We are traveling on a slippery learning curve that can trip us up at any given moment. The thoughts that flood through our minds directly affect and create the world of existence around us.

Many people are wasting precious life energy making a living and are consumed by working in order to achieve and attain more and more. In our society we have created a system for exchanging our life energy for survival. There are valid things which we do indeed need in order to endure. These include food, air, water and shelter.

Our emotional body desires love and the formation of relationships. Our intellectual layer wishes to learn and in turn share our experiences and insights. The existential thinkers have pondered this for centuries exploring the higher states of consciousness.

It is a fact that we must meet our basic needs in such a way that we are really feeding only those that truly make us happy. In order to really see this, we must track our earning and spending over the course of six months and then calculate how much we need to exist.

Most of us do not actually sit down and ask ourselves "how much do I need?" and most of our decisions are ego based. Rather than having a focused idea of what we need and what is really making us happy, our ego-minds are continually moving the guidepost, causing constant fluctuation to our paths. This is a great part of what drives many of us to strive, achieve and obtain. Even when we are conscious and aware of this behavior, we still want more stuff.

We must get a clear view of what is essential and what is not important. One of the tricks to understanding where you are is to stay focused on just this. The moment we begin to cross compare is when we tilt the scales and blur out of focus.

Those of the great earners and achievers, who are indeed happy, give ninety percent of what they obtain away. This is due to the fact that what we receive when we volunteer is satisfying. When giving in selfless service we must offer energy with absolutely no expectation in any way.

There was a woman we knew who came to stay with us at an ashram for a three month commitment of Seva. As we got to know her and watched her, we were overtaken by the compassionate and loving energy she placed into every single chore and activity.

She was from a foreign country and did not speak the language but this did not throw her off at all. If she was washing a humongous cooking pot after dinner, or sweeping a pathway, she always seemed not only peaceful but genuinely grateful. There was not an ounce of ego involved in her actions. If she was asked to work during a gathering or missed an event, she took this all in stride. The more we grew to know her, the more we were touched by her gentle spirit of acceptance. She did not expect an outcome and it was obvious that every molecule of her being was in service to the community.

When we learn to act in this method of true selfless service, we begin to generate a sense of peace and love in our energy fields. Ultimately this brings a deep-felt sense of contentment. This satisfaction is a state where we experience "aha" moments of blissful energy.

Performing seva can happen at anytime, anywhere and at any level of volunteering. We do not need to cloister at an ashram or hide away. The key to getting this right is that we must do it with no ego-based expectation.

FLOWERING

Opening up to joy and bliss by activating prana[22], then allowing it to move us

The Importance of Artistic and Creative Expression

The happiest people are the ones who partake in daily expressive arts. This can be visual art, dance, music, writing and any type of performance that quenches the thirst for beauty and expression. Emotional attraction and aesthetic pleasure come from many creative sources in art and nature. Somewhere along the way in our society the idea of desire became misconstrued. In the ancient east yearning is an essential value. The fact that sensory enjoyment is a natural and healthy state is taught to children when they are very young.

During the course of human development, when we move from egotistic behavior to knowledge of self and happiness within, we go through various levels. Flowering of consciousness, activating our prana and releasing it from energetic blocks begins to occur spontaneously and effortlessly. Removing obstacles in different layers of our existence leads us to experience free flowing energy. This connects us to our higher self and our true nature which is joy, bliss and happiness and is a cathartic experience.

The art of relaxation at will is extremely important. Mind, body and breath are interconnected to each other. When mind is quiet and calm,

---

22 **Prana** प्राण *prANa* Breath, the energy of the life force.

breath slows down and body becomes relaxed. When body is relaxed, breath becomes quiet and mind becomes calm. You can enter the state of higher self—true nature—through techniques such as breathing practices and the deep relaxation of the body through a myriad of creative visualization techniques.

Creativity

We are creative beings. When we are children we know we are creative at a deep inner level. We need very little encouragement to express ourselves. We sing and dance, draw and tell stories by nature. We do it purely for the joy of making others happy from a level of profound inner knowing. This is a birthright that early in our existence we all find easy to express.

When it comes to creativity children are naturals. They can animate any object and give it a story and purpose. These are integral skills to infuse into our energetic bodies and help to create happiness as adults. When children are involved in a task they are fully present and one hundred percent engaged. This ability to be mindful is a great part of what generates happiness.

The act of creativity is truly for the sake of the immersion in action. There is no ideal set as to the outcome. Artistic expression is the process and not the product. The older we become, the more important it is to be creative. The happiest elders we know have creative outlets. These become more and more important as we age.

As children we were not expected to explain ourselves when playing—we just played for the pure joy of it. We knew at an intuitive level when we were being given good attention and we received a lot of unconditional love. Our schedules were more steady and regular and this created an ease for sleeping, eating and digesting. We loved to smile and laugh.

Laughter is great fertilizer to urge the budding and opening of happiness. It is known that laughing helps to reduce anxiety and stress and fosters a positive attitude and a feeling of happiness. The health benefits of laughter are extensive. It is beneficial to the cardiovascular system and helps to reduce blood pressure.

Here is something you can try:

There are many ways to get yourself giggling. Explore everything from joke telling, to comedy movies and books. You can even join a laughter club.

LETTING GO
Release and Surrender

The concept of attachment versus non-attachment can be confusing. This is due to the element of surrender needed to become fully unattached. We can get caught in a sticky web of confusion over the idea of surrender. Even if we do grasp what this is all about, it can still be challenging to put the concept into action. It is easy for us to become stuck in an early phase of letting go or find it difficult to launch into the non-doing state. Sometimes we want to push through to the final chapter; other times, we cling to the patterns of our current situation.

When presented with the need to really let go and the ability to see imminent endpoints, an array of emotions kick in. Perhaps we can see all the signs telling us to move on and can even watch ourselves making decisions. We may have a deep knowing that what we are considering is not for the highest good of ourselves and the greater collective. What is it that keeps us from true surrender?

Consider a caterpillar and its journey to becoming a butterfly.

A Caterpillar's Story of Letting Go
One day, in the bright sunshine, a group of caterpillars crawled on a wild plant, munching on leaves. Though each was consumed by the perception of hunger, each had a running inner monologue.

One little caterpillar thought, *"This leaf is delicious. I wish it would last forever."*

A second caterpillar murmured in-between mouthfuls,

"What will happen when there are no more leaves to eat?"

Another doubted the brilliance of his stripes and felt inferior to his caterpillar buddies. In spite of these thoughts, the force of their inner need to feed kept them going. As the wind gently caressed the edge of the forest where the feast continued and the sun sailed past its highpoint at noon, one caterpillar's voice broke the silence as she called out,

"I cannot go on. I feel I must leave this situation here and now!"

Another responded sadly,
"Don't go. I will miss you terribly."

A great debate ensued, and the caterpillars began to argue the situation. Some had issues of self-esteem, while others disputed the same leaf as personal territory.

A wise caterpillar shattered the mayhem and commanded,
"Let us stop this feeding and frenzy of thought. It is now time for us to transform."

A small curious caterpillar crawled toward the sage and asked,
"What is it that we must do?"

"It is time for us to find stillness so that we can change. End the suffering of the mind and thoughts by finding a tranquil and sturdy place to wrap yourself in a cocoon of quiet. Just find a spot on a branch and surrender. This way, your body and your true nature can take over. You do not need to do anything."

"I am afraid," the little caterpillar choked.

"I understand," came the response from the older caterpillar as he began to shed his skin and still himself in a meditative slumber. "Just let go, little one," he added.

It takes a lot of willpower and trust to surrender to the many challenges we are faced with in life at all levels. Fortunately there is help to guide us.

Surrender and Non-attachment

The mind likes to step in and try to confuse us. Problems occur when we get lost in the mind-stuff and our thoughts. These tangle us in disturbance and chaos. The constant river of thought causes us to develop attachment to the external world in the form of people, places, or things. The perceptive individual mind becomes overactive and reactive, and this leads to suffering when the material trappings are gone.

Through the practice of meditation and finding the witness state, we are able to back up from the mind and give it space. Once a perspective view is found, we can then tune into the sensation that we are not this mind, nor these thoughts.

When the idea of non-attachment is presented, it immediately stirs the mind and heart with fear and anxiety. The inner child screams, "No!" We can surrender only at the point when we become completely unattached. This non-attachment must be at all levels of existence. It is important to realize that the mind itself is only an instrument, just like our hands, legs, eyes, and ears. The mind's job is thinking. It is an important tool needed to interact with the world outside, but it is not who we really are.

We must realize that everything in the universe is impermanent. All things in life are cyclical. They have a beginning, middle, and endpoint. Therefore they are surely going to perish one day. Things come into being, they are born, they stay for a while, and then, when the time is right, they are gone. When we really embrace this it is easier to become non-attached.

In a millisecond we believe we must be prepared to give up everything and run away from the material world into the forest. There is no need to leave society and become an ascetic, though some have solved this conundrum by doing so. The natural habitat is not the actual woods but the tranquil state of meditation. When we tune into the idea of non-attachment we are able to reach an inner knowing, and that it is a necessary part of our true nature.

Stand on the bank of a river and watch it flow. Notice how it is letting go of the water, which is there in front of you. Moment to moment the water changes and the river brings in new water. This is continuous. In the autumn, deciduous trees shed their leaves, preparing for a slumber. The sap of a tree dives deep into the roots, and this allows the tree to be still and resting in a form of meditation. This is followed by an invitation to embrace spring with fresh new growth. It is important for us to grasp this as a necessary daily need. The only thing preventing our understanding of this about ourselves is our sense of insecurity.

The Buddha shared teachings about this in the four noble truths. His core teachings emphasized these concepts in an effort to awaken us to the perception of non-attachment.

The four noble truths of the Buddha

1. The truth of human life is suffering.
2. The cause of suffering is our attachment to what is pleasurable and

our aversion to pain as a result of our belief system and our attachment to people, places, or things that are inherently impermanent.

3. There is a way out of this suffering. The truth of cessation to suffering is through non-attachment to our beliefs—our likes and dislikes—and people, places, and things that are inherently impermanent.

4. Nonattachment is achieved through the eightfold path that includes meditation, discipline, correct behavior, compassion, and truthfulness.

Many masters have shared an ancient Zen story of two monks in order to explain this concept. Here is our version of the story.

"One day an older monk and a younger monk were walking down a quiet dirt road, returning to their monastery. The older monk, who was walking ahead, came to the bank of a river. As he looked toward the water where they would cross, he saw a beautiful young woman wearing an elaborately embroidered silk dress. Her expression was troubled.

"The elder monk quickly looked away and decided to ignore her in full honor of his vows, which commanded that he not have contact with members of the opposite sex. The young lady grimaced and sighed watching the old man paying her no attention. He gave a wide berth to where the woman sat and quietly made his way down the bank and across the river. Once on the other side, he began to head for home.

"Upon reaching the top of the opposite bank, he looked back across the water to see where his younger companion was. The elder monk was horrified to see the young monk carrying the woman across the river on his shoulders. He watched as the younger monk let her down gently and bowed in farewell. The younger monk then continued on his way to catch up with his senior companion, who was now waiting a little bit down the road in the shade of a tree.

"The two monks continued on, walking in silence for quite some time, winding their way up a stony path to the monastery. When they were just outside the ornate gates of the hermitage, the elder monk scolded the younger monk.

'What you did was not good! You have broken our rules! We are not supposed to have such contact with women.' His face wrinkled in disdain as he continued, 'Even beyond this, you carried her on your back!'

"The younger monk paused and looked at the ground beneath his feet for a moment. He then looked his superior in the eyes and said,

'I left her on the bank of the river. Apparently, you are still carrying her.'"

This story is a wonderful example of how we become attached to our belief system. These unique energetic organizations of thought outlive the physical body. They are carried through the path of lifetimes until we come to terms with them and complete the evolutionary lesson. The Main Obstacles Upon the Path to Happiness:

Ignorance is a veil that prevents us from knowing the true nature of self.

Egotism causes us to be lost in the material world. This produces a craving for power and a need for validation.

Attachment is a result of unreal belief systems and a desire to attain things that are impermanent.

Aversion is a belief that that we must form opinions of likes and dislikes. The only neutral point is true detachment.

Clinging to life creates a fear of death. A better way is to live each moment as if it is the last, be grateful for all good, and give love.

We want and desire and aspire toward a utopic ideal of what we believe is perfect in the pursuit of happiness. As a society, we spend billions on improving the look and shape of the bodies in which we reside. This far outweighs the amount of effort placed in changing our thoughts and patterns.

It is a known fact that people who seemingly have less in the way of possessions are statistically happier. This does not mean one must give away everything, but it is proven that when a large portion of what we accrue is given away, we are indeed a great deal happier. Keep in mind, it is as important to remain safe and secure as it is imperative to stay out of the feelings of fear. Fear is the antithesis of love, and love is the reason we are here.

The true desire to change comes only when we are entirely fed up and completely give up and let go. This is how and when we are able to come to a state of total surrender. To be in this state does not mean we do not love people, places, or things, nor does it mean that we are not grateful for what we have drawn into our lives. We must come to the realization that the material world and its array of objects are not our reasons to be. Understanding this truth and wisdom helps us to let our emotional clinginess go. In order to fill a perceived gap we must give ourselves over to love and acceptance. Love is the utmost important feeling and gift we have to share with the world. When we choose to love, infinite possibilities present themselves.

The Magic of Sleep

Every night when we drift off in slumber, the mind has an opportunity to disconnect from the objective world. This is when the computer processing of the electrical mind can clear the fragments of the day.

Sleep is a natural state we must reach each night for rest and rejuvenation. In the peaceful domain of sleep we return to our true nature. While sleeping, we are not attached to anything. There are no possessions, no relationships, no problems, and no ego. If we can practice non-attachment while we are sleeping, we can practice it during the day, as well. Many people are plagued by the inability to sleep. We are wired in such a way that it is impossible to detach from the material world in the waking state. This is the reason it is difficult for many to surrender, release, and relax.

There is a plethora of reasons as to what causes the inability to sleep, ranging from lack of sunshine and poor health practices to sleep environment, diet, and emotional stress. In addition, those who do not have the ability to completely disconnect from the object world around us find it very difficult to reach the calm and necessary place to let go and relax. In order to do this we must release the exterior world. When the internal world and the external world are toxic, we need help to let go and find balance. The first step is emotional detoxification.

Health at All Levels

In order to reach an optimum state of being, we must learn to cleanse and balance at the three levels of body, mind, and spirit. Then we are in a state of Svasthya[23], or health. The process of a Panchakarma is used as a vehicle to return to the self. If we focus only on the mind by means of talk therapy and psychology, there is no way to return to the source. Without an optimal state of health, the effects are temporary.

The art of cellular detoxification utilized in Ayurveda known as Panchakarma translates as "five actions." This fivefold technique helps to give the body, mind, and spirit a chance to rebalance. Toxins accumulate in the body, creating stickiness as a result of unprocessed emotions. In order to begin to process this emotional toxicity, we must find a way to take ownership and accept it as a part of who we are. The key to handling this is to not become attached to it. Instead, we must witness it as if it is a separate thing. Then we can give it space to be and become non-reactive. In the witness state, we can create space for it.

---

23 **Svasthya** स्वस्थय *svAsthya* A state of being established in the self, signifying health at all levels in emotional, social, physical and energetic producing harmony.

This, in turn, allows it to pass.

Addiction is present when we are stuck and not processing emotions while letting them control us. Unprocessed emotions and behavioral patterns can be passed through families and generations. Therefore, we can inherit the propensity for behavioral patterns as well as physical genetic configurations. As long as we are able to move in the direction of joy, we are progressing on the right course. Many good ideas and ways of instilling change can become habit forming. This in turn can become positive habit.

There are many schools of thought and practice in the realm of Yoga to help us detoxify the spirit, mind, and body. Some use sound and repetition, while others use silence and stillness. There is no right or wrong way.

The ability to let go is easier with the utilization of sound, exercise, and creative expression. This can be dancing, singing, drawing, or writing. We can also find release in shopping, receiving a massage, connecting with nature, or helping others through selfless service and volunteering. Once freed, we can celebrate and experience happiness.

Seasonal Changes

Summer is the season in which Pitta humor accumulates in the body. Fall is the season when Vata accumulates in the body. Spring is the season when Kapha accumulates in the body. Panchakarma, performed during specific seasonal changes, yields the best results by removing aggravated humors and thus acts as a preventive of disease.

Panchakarma to remove physical and mental Ama is especially valuable in creating a state of well-being both at a physical and the mental layer of our beings. Once the physical Ama is removed, humors can flow uninterrupted through the channels of the body to bring in appropriate nutrition and eliminate unwanted waste products from the tissues. When mental Ama is removed, there is free flow of Prana that opens and balances all of the Chakras. This creates homeostasis. Prana, along with choiceless awareness and consciousness, eventually becomes the source of all healing and prevention in Ayurveda.

Panchakarma is a precious and needed gift to create good health and is used as a vehicle to get back to the self and to the consciousness. If we only detoxify the mind and body without a way to return to the source, the effects are only temporary. Source, consciousness—the true self—is primary and is the true healer for the vehicle of Prana. Svasthya is being established in the self. Without a state of Svasthya, health does not happen. Happiness is this state of health.

The set of procedures that follow the main treatments of Panchakarma, called post-Panchakarma therapies, are aimed at assisting the body in the re-establishment of a healthy metabolism and immune system. The body is in a sensitive, somewhat vulnerable state after treatment. If these post-treatment procedures are neglected, the digestion may not normalize and the production of toxins would continue. Therefore, following a Panchakarma program, it is advised to keep eating light, nourishing foods, such as mung dal soup and rice, and then gradually adding vegetables and other foods. It is also recommended to slowly and gradually return to regular activities. In this way we are able to avoid taxing the nervous system.

The lifestyle program that should be adopted at this time to support the Panchakarma treatment is a daily routine. The Ayurvedic clinician gives specific guidelines for this as well as additional seasonal guidelines and recommendations. They also provide the client with rasayanas[24], which are herbal and mineral preparations with specific rejuvenating effects on body and mind. Rasayanas increase vitality and energy. They nourish and rejuvenate the entire organism, and thus are an important part of the post-Panchakarma procedures.

A Personal Story of a Client and His Experience of Finding Ayurveda

"I am a thirty-six year old man, and I met Dr. Jain about four years

---

24 **Rasayana** रसायन *rasAyana* Literally meaning path of essence and relating to an elixir.

ago. Prior to meeting him I had heard of Ayurveda but didn't really know anything about it. I had been struggling with addiction since I was a teenager. My blood pressure and my cholesterol were high and I was diagnosed as being pre-diabetic. The doctor I was seeing at the time told me I needed to be on medication for diabetes. In addition I was taking anti-depressants, attention-deficit-disorder medication, and suboxone—a drug that helps ease you off opiates.

"It is really interesting to look back at how my life made a sudden change. It is easy to say I wasn't really doing so well in any aspect of my health or life at that time. I wasn't looking for Ayurveda or Dr. Jain—at least I don't think I was.

"I went to a weekend retreat at a Yoga institute for an addiction workshop. It combined addiction counseling, education, group work—all the things you would expect at something like this, but in addition they were also teaching energy healing and yoga. Before that weekend when I had my first encounter with the guru, my perception of yoga was that it was pretty much something that women did. It just looked like stretching to me. After hearing the guru speak about yoga, I knew I had stumbled upon something really special. My perspective on yoga, addiction, spirituality, and life were shifted spontaneously.

"At the end of the weekend I met the guru's son and was offered a possible job working with Dr. Jain as a therapist for Panchakarma. I honestly couldn't believe he was serious because of the way I saw myself at the time. Rather than sharing my doubt, I said I would love to work with him and that it would be amazing. I went home never expecting to hear from him, but to my surprise I received a call about a week later to meet with Dr. Jain.

"On my way there I was so nervous. I had only been a massage therapist for short time, and most interviews I'd had with doctors had not gone very well. This made me anxious and uneasy. When I arrived and met him, I was greeted with such graciousness that I felt instantly at ease—far more than I had expected to be. He hired me and suggested a couple of books to read about Ayurveda before I was scheduled to begin working in a few weeks.

"When I began, I weighed one-hundred-eighty-five pounds and felt ill in all aspects of my life—physically, energetically, and emotionally. Nothing had felt right in my relationships, with my mental state, nor spiritually. My wife had recently left me and kept the house. I have two daughters that I was only getting to see infrequently. I felt so miserable; I didn't think they should be around me.

"I was full of negativity. This manifested as shame, guilt, blame, and anger. Somehow, at this turning point, I began to feel something different. I experienced so much gratitude for this opportunity and welcomed it with a great deal of excitement. This gave me hope and showed me that my life was not over, but rather it was shifting. I had the sense that I was renewed and that this was a great opportunity to begin a new chapter.

"I started my new job and right away felt like I was a part of something meaningful. I felt welcome. I knew right away I had found my teachers and was given the opportunity to begin a new kind of life. I began working as a therapist for Panchakarma and listening to Dr. Jain give lectures each night during the programs. This and the books I was reading gave me a new understanding of the body and how life and energy work. Together these helped me to quit my one pack a day smoking habit and inspired me to begin practicing yoga and meditation. The simple tips I picked up like not having ice cold drinks, not eating unless I feel hunger, and to stop eating before I feel full made huge changes in the way I felt. I spontaneously became a vegetarian and life started to feel right.

"I decided to stop taking all of my medication and see if yoga and Ayurveda were all I needed. I eagerly experimented with each new technique I learned. I tried the idea of having all six tastes in each meal. I gained an understanding of my Dosha type, which is Pitta, and got an Ayurvedic cookbook. Each day I made adjustments and changes to my diet and lifestyle in accordance with my understanding of what would help to bring me back into balance.

"Each time I returned to work as a massage therapist in a Panchakarma program, I would continue to gain more knowledge from

Dr. Jain's lectures, and I listened to the guru's talks every morning before work. I practiced and implemented everything I was learning. It was easy to do because I was feeling and noticing how my life and body were being affected, which was truly amazing. I shed thirty pounds right away without even thinking about losing weight. It just happened from making subtle changes. I'm now the same weight I was in high school. After seeing how much this wisdom was helping me, I decided to start taking courses on Yoga, meditation, and Ayurveda.

"It has been almost five years since the day I met Dr. Jain and I can honestly say that my life has been changed from top to bottom. I am still off all medication. I no longer have issues with addiction, and my relationships have all improved, especially with myself. Most importantly, I'm happy.

"This was all possible just by understanding some basic principles of Ayurveda and Yoga and then, of course, applying them to my life and making them my daily practice. I feel, even beyond the physical changes, the most important addition has been meditation and self-study."

Unfolding Happiness

REJUVENATION
The Continuum of Re-seeding

Our True Nature Is Joy, Bliss, and Happiness

In Ayurveda, there is a substance known as Ojas. This is essential life energy. Ojas is a wholesome biochemical constituent that nourishes all tissues and provides immunity to the physical body and the mind. It is produced as a result of perfect digestion, absorption, and assimilation of nutrients in the tissues.

Ojas is considered, in Ayurveda, to be the purest substance in the universe. It is omnipresent in humans and is responsible for higher states of consciousness. The presence of Ojas brings purity of thought and provides the necessary environment to be in a state of perfect health, happiness, and harmony.

When Ojas is in abundance, we experience positive feelings like love and joy. Our bodies have a greater ease of immunity, and this in turn increases our potential for longevity. Ojas is a key component. With a greater presence of Ojas, our minds function more smoothly. We experience an increase in our level of intelligence and feel more creative. Our memory increases, and this in turn brings us into a higher level of happiness and bliss.

Dynamics that disturb our levels of Ojas are excessive worry and any sensation of unhappiness. Injury at any level upsets this delicate substance. Emotional unhappiness from grief, anger, and excessive thinking disrupts the equilibrium just as the physical pain of hunger, over-exertion, and more intense hurt, like the loss of blood, can.

Positivity in feelings, speech, and behavior, and love, joy, and appreciation produce more Ojas and better immunity. Our conduct can have a health-promoting influence on body biochemistry. These behaviors are love, compassion, and nonviolence in thought, speech, and action known as ahimsa[25]. Other integral positive acts include cleanliness, charity, and reverence to one's external as well as internal teacher, moderation, self-control, and simplicity.

When Ojas is in abundance, our reproductive tissues work at the most optimum level. Ojas is a biochemical substance believed to have a profound influence on the quality of mental and emotional life as well as physical health. In modern science terminology, Ojas might be equivalent to neuropeptides from the hypothalamus, which are perceived to have identical effects.

One of the most important ways to improve digestion, immunity, and Ojas is to do regular detoxification therapies. Once the impurities are removed from the body, cells and tissues return to an optimum state, creating ideal digestion and production of Ojas. A regular practice of meditation is an essential component of any rejuvenation program. Yogic breathing exercises and postures energize and balance the mind-body physiology. The daily oil massage assists in the elimination of toxins and releases neuropeptides from the skin. Nourishing and supportive relationships provide the right medium in which rejuvenation can take place. Living in the present moment in all aspects of our lives helps us to metabolize the sensory inputs and creates a balanced, happy, and joyous state.

Adopting a meditation practice and taking time to connect with nature is vitally important. Through these simple practices, we nurture an awakening from the unconscious state that Yoga teaches us is like a delusive dream. To consciously awaken and be established in the self

---

25 **Ahimsa** अहिंसा *ahiMsA* Nonviolence. Abstinence from injury; harmlessness, not causing of pain to any living creature in thought, word, or deed at any time.

leads us on a journey to enlightenment.

Spiritual dissidence occurs when our inner world meets the outer world. Ego is the veil that has to be penetrated in order for this to happen. We have all had intense wake-up calls that profoundly show us when the true ego is at work. This changes our awareness as to what is more important with regard to health and happiness.

When we learn to read signs and patterns of obstructions and flow, we are able to tune into the subtleties of how the universe works. The result is an ease and spontaneous fulfillment of desires. These unfold and reveal newfound health, happiness, and contentment. We must learn to let the heart, rather than the head, lead us through decision-making and find the place of acceptance and happiness with the way the world is around us and how we are. It is in this acceptance and realization that happiness blossoms.

The science of happiness teaches us that it is more important to pray for being happy rather than for someone or something which will make us happy. Shopping and spending are temporary fixes and create a state of happiness that is rented but never owned. When the ego structure is dismantled, happiness comes from deep inside and is no longer dependent on external sources.

True happiness embraces all that is. We let go of the fears that surround loss and death. We wake up from the delusional dream of society and understand that death and the act of letting go are to be accepted as a part of the natural continuum of existence. This in turn helps us to understand that we are always connected and that the idea of separation is an illusion. This awakening brings us to a renewed place where we can begin to live our lives in a vibrant, healthy, and happy manner.

CONCLUSION

Most people erroneously believe that happiness comes from achieving success in professional and personal relationships. When what we have is ignored and we are not grateful, but rather strive to satisfy every desire that enters our field of awareness, it is easy to become confused when the outcome is a feeling of unhappiness.

Our view of the world is an important factor. Do we witness life as a glass half empty or half full? An optimist enjoys life as full and rich with gifts, while a pessimist complains about lack and only focuses on what is missing. It is therefore essential to learn to be more optimistic and grateful for what we have.

We, as human beings, prefer activities that are motivated by the avoidance of pain and yearning. We rearrange the world around us so that we do not feel discomfort and instead continuously seek out joy. Unfortunately, the external world changes constantly and therefore our happiness can be transitory.

It is a fact that most of our unhappiness can be traced to our preoccupation with our view of the physical body and our feelings regarding our expectation of how the world should be. When we are able to let go of the belief that sensory pleasures are responsible for our happiness, we rediscover the happy state within us that is always there, regardless of the variables in the external world.

A wise Persian proverb states, "I complained that I had no shoes until I met a man who had no feet."

Indeed, happiness is a state of mind. Through the practice of meditation we are able to learn and understand that sensory input and physical objects only activate a temporary state of happiness. We believe it is possible to arrive at an awareness of this without going through suffering or loss. The intention is better set on self-observance and giving gratitude. This helps to keep our emotions and desires in balance.

Happiness is a state of being that is already present within us. It is easy to become confused, thinking that being healthy leads to happiness, or that people, places, and things can bring it to us. The external world can trigger this state for a short time, but it is not long lasting. The ability of outside influences to create happiness decreases over time.

Happiness, which is our true state, needs to be gently unfolded. This unfoldment comes as a result of our awakening to what is real and what is unreal. When we are happy, we experience synchronistic success in every field of life automatically and spontaneously.

We wish you infinite happiness!

SANSKRIT GLOSSARY

Agni अग्नि *agni* The Lord of fire as well as fire itself. The digestive fire.

Ahimsa अहिंसा *ahiMsA* Nonviolence. Abstinence from injury; harmlessness; not causing pain to any living creature in thought, word, or deed at any time.

Akasha आकाश *AkAsha* Space, sky ether.

Ama आम *Ama* Undigested, uncooked.

Ananda आनन्द *Ananda* Bliss, joy, delight, happiness.

Anuloma Viloma अनुलोम विलोम *anuloma viloma* A practice of alternate nostril breathing a type of **Nadi Shodhana** नाडी शोधन *nADI shodhana* which helps to bring balance to the nadis.

Artha अर्थ *artha* Purpose, motive, meaning, cause, wealth, economy.

Asana आसन *Asana* A body position, typically associated with the practice of Yoga originally identified as the mastery of sitting still. In the Yoga sutras of Patanjali it is suggested that asana is "to be seated in a position that is firm, but relaxed" for extended, or timeless periods.

Avidya अविद्या *avidyA* Ignorance, spiritual ignorance, non-existence, unwise, foolish.

Ayurveda आयुर्वेद *Ayurveda* Ayurveda is the traditional healing modality of the Vedic culture from India, said to be 2000 to 5000 years old. Ayurveda literally translates as "the wisdom of life" or "the knowledge of longevity."

Bhagavad Gita भगवद्गीता *bhagavadgItA* A 700-verse Hindu scripture that is part of the epic Mahabharata. It is classified as Smriti स्मृति *smR^iti* and Krishna's song.

Brahman ब्रह्मन् *brahman* The one supreme, Universal Spirit.

Chit चित् *cit* Understand, comprehend, observe.

Chitta चित्त *citta* Thought.

Dharma धर्म *dharma* Nature, manner, those behaviors considered necessary for the maintenance of the natural order of things.

Dosha दोष *doSha* A body humor.

Guna गुण *guNa* Attribute or quality pertaining to nature.

Jala जल *jala* Water.

Jyotish ज्योतिस् *jyotish* Light as brightness and as the divine principle of life and source of intelligence. The science and movement of the heavenly bodies.

Kapalabhati कपालभाति *kapAlbhAti* Skull shining or skull cleansing. A breathing practice.

Kapha कफ *kapha* The humor of earth and water.

Karma कर्म *karma* Action.

Krishna कृष्ण *krSNa* Literally dark, black or dark blue which represents space. The eighth avatar of Lord Vishnu. Traditionally attributed with the authorship of the Bhagavad Gita.

Mahabharata महाभारत *mahAbArata* One of the two major epics written in Sanskrit.

Mantra मन्त्र *mantra* A sound, a syllable, a word or group of words possessing transformative power. The words and use are particular to each school of thought and sacred lineage.

Nadi नाडी *nADI* River, flowing water, tube, pipe. The ancient texts say there are 72,000 Nadis in the human body.

Nadi Shodhana नाडी शोधन *nADI shodhana* Chanel clearing breath. A form of Pranayama that helps to clear out blocked energy and calms the mind.

Nidra निद्रा *nidrA* Literally, sleep. A deep state of complete relaxation in meditation. Yogic sleep.

Ojas ओजस् *ojas* Primal vigor. Bodily strength, vigor, splendor, luster. The subtle energy of water as our vital energy reserve.

Panchakarma पञ्चकर्म *pañchakarma* Literally, five actions.

Patanjali पतञ्जलि *patanjali* Name of a philosopher who was also a physician who lived 150 BCE.

Pitta पित्त *pitta* The humor of fire and water.

Prakriti प्रकृति *prakR^iti* Nature. The basic nature of intelligence by which the Universe exists and functions.

Prana प्राण *prANa* Breath, the energy of the life force.

Pranayama प्राणायाम *prANAyAma* Suspending the breath. Modulating breath.

Prithvi पृथ्वी *pRthvI* Earth. The element of earth.

Ramayana रामायण *rAmAyaNa* An ancient epic written in Sanskrit depicting Rama's journey. **Rama** राम *rAma* is an avatar of the Hindu God **Vishnu** विष्णु *viShNu*.

Rasayana रसायन *rasAyana* Literally meaning path of essence and relating to an elixir.

Santosha संतोष *saMtoSa* Contentedness.

Sat सत् *sat* True, truth.

Sattvic सात्त्विक *sAttva* Relating to the quality of **Sattva**. Guna of intelligence, purity, existence, reality.

Seva सेवा *sevA* Service.

Sutra सूत्र *sUtra* Thread formula, string or discourse.

Smriti स्मृति *smR^iti* A whole body of codes of law as handed down memoriter or by tradition.

Svasthya स्वस्थय *svAsthya* A state of being established in the self, signifying health at all levels in emotional, social, physical and energetic producing harmony.

Vata वात *vAta* The humor of air and space.

Vayu वायु *vAyu* Vital air.

Vedas वेदा: *vedaH* True or sacred knowledge. Texts originating in ancient India. The oldest scriptures of Hinduism.

Vikriti विकृति *vikR^iti* Change, disease, modification.

Vishnu विष्णु *vishNu* The all preserving essence of all beings in the Trimurti.

Vritti वृत्ति *vR^itti* Frequent repetition of the same.

Yoga योग *yoga* A physical, mental and spiritual discipline originating in ancient India.

Yoga Chitta Vritti Nirodha योग: चित्त वृत्ति निरोध: *yogaH chitta vR^itti nirodhaH* Yoga is a set of contextual directions to individuals, for the goal of refining and regulating psycho-spiritual propensities.

APPENDIX I
Learn Your Dosha

The Dosha Quiz to Determine
Prakriti Mind-Body Constitution

There are two parts to this questionnaire. The first part determines your unique constitution or *Prakriti*.

Answer the questions in Part I as to how you have been all your life, on both a physical as well as a psychological basis. If one answer alone does not feel like a description of you, then you can use two answers for that particular question. Add up all of the columns. The column that has the highest sum denotes your constitution.

Part I

Frame	☐	I have small bones and am thin and slender with a slight build and fairly narrow hips and shoulders. Some would call me unusually tall or short.	☐	I have medium bones, am of average height, and a symmetrical and well-proportioned build.	☐	I have a sturdy heavier build and am of average height. Weight
Weight	☐	I have a tendency to lose weight.	☐	I find it easy to gain weight.	☐	I gain weight easily but have difficulty losing it.
Eyes	☐	My eyes are relatively small and some would say my gaze is active or curious.	☐	I have medium sized eyes and most would say I have a penetrating gaze.	☐	I have relatively large eyes and most would say my gaze is soft and pleasant.

Complexion	☐ My skin is dry, rough and thin. I tan easily without burning. I have a few moles that are dark in color.	☐ My skin is warm and reddish. I burn easily in the sun. I have many moles and freckles that are brownish red.	☐ My skin is soft, thick, moist and smooth. I can tan after long exposure. I have a few light moles and some white blotches.
Hair	☐ My hair tends to be dry, brittle, scanty and curly, sometimes frizzy. My eyelashes are thin.	☐ My hair is fine and straight, and blond, red, or prematurely gray in color. I have a tendency toward baldness or thinning hair.	☐ My hair is soft, thick, and abundant.
Joints	☐ My joints are thin, prominent, and tend to crack. My veins and tendons are noticeable.	☐ My joints are loose and flexible. My veins and tendons are prominent.	☐ My joints are large and padded. My veins and tendons are not prominent.
Menses (for women)	☐ My cycle is irregular. My flow is scanty and dark.	☐ My Cycle is regular. My flow is intense and red.	☐ My cycle is average and the flow is light.
Appetite	☐ My appetite varies. I like to eat frequently though sometimes I forget to eat.	☐ I have a moderate to strong appetite. I like to have regular meals on time and don't like to miss meals.	☐ I like to eat but am often not really hungry. I can miss a meal with little effect.

Food Preferences	☐ I love salads and crunchy snacks.	☐ I love spicy, hot, and oily foods.	☐ I enjoy sweet and starchy foods.
Sex Drive	☐ I am easily aroused and quickly satiated.	☐ I can be romantic and passionate and have a strong sex drive, with controlled passion and average stamina.	☐ I am slow to be aroused, but am deeply involved and have good stamina.
Sleep Pattern	☐ I am a light sleeper with a tendency to awaken easily.	☐ I am a moderately sound sleeper and need less than eight hours.	☐ I sleep deeply and am often find it difficult to awaken.
Body Temperature	☐ My hands and feet are cold. I prefer a warm environment.	☐ I am usually warm and prefer a cooler environment	☐ I am adaptable to most temperatures but dislike cold.
Temperament	☐ I am lively and enthusiastic by nature and like to change.	☐ I am purposeful and intense. I like to convince. I am competitive, enjoy challenges, and like to be in command. I've been called a natural leader. Some find me pushy, stubborn, or opinionated.	☐ I tend to be easy going, relaxed, and accepting.

The second part of the questionnaire determines imbalances, or *Vikriti*. Mark the correct answer to each of the following questions. Answer these questions according to what is most true of you now. Score your answers by using the following scale in order to indicate how well each statement applies to your life experiences over the past few months. Each "Never" is 1 point, an "Occasionally" is 3 points, and "Always" is 5 points.

Part II

Vata Assessment

Vata score: Never x1, Occasionally x3, Always x5	Never	Occasionally	Always
I have been feeling nervous, fearful, panicky anxious or frantic.			
I have been having difficulty falling asleep or have been awakening easily.			
I have been acting impulsively or inconsistently.			
I have been more forgetful than usual.			
I have been feeling restless or uneasy. My skin is dry and easily chapped.			
I am suffering from dry, hard stools, constipation, and gas or bloating, or I am having loose stools when emotionally upset.			
I am becoming intolerant of cold.			
My daily schedule of eating meals, going to sleep, or waking up has been inconsistent from day to day.			
Total Vata scores			

Pitta Assessment

Pitta score: Never x1, Occasionally x3, Always x5	Never	Occasionally	Always
I have been feeling irritable or impatient.			
I have a red, inflamed, or burning rash, acne, cold sores or fever blisters.			
I have been feeling critical and intolerant of others.			
I enjoy spicy foods but they have been causing heartburn or acid reflux.			
I feel like I am overheated or having hot flashes.			
My bowels are loose or I am having two to three BMs a day.			
I have been feeling frustrated, irritable, or angry.			
I have been behaving compulsively and find it difficult to stop once I have started working on a project.			
My eyes are red, inflamed, or sensitive to light.			
I expect perfection of myself and others.			
Total Pitta scores			

Kapha Assessment

Kapha score: Never x1, Occasionally x3, Always x5	Never	Occasionally	Always
I have excessive mucus in my body or sinuses or lung congestion.			
I have been dealing with conflict by withdrawing.			
I have been accumulating more clutter than usual in my life.			
I am overweight.			
I am stubborn and resistant to change.			
I am having difficulty leaving a job, a relationship, or a situation even though it is not nourishing me.			
I have been spending more time in watching rather than participating in athletic activity.			
It is difficult for me to wake up in the morning even if I sleep deeply for eight to ten hours.			
I am prone to excessive emotional eating, especially of sweet, heavy foods.			
My bowels movements are slow, sticky, and sluggish or feel incomplete.			
Total Kapha scores			

Totals	Never	Occasionally	Always
Total for Part I			
Total for Part II			
Grand Total of Parts I and II			
***Prakriti*, My Constitution** Any humor in Part I that is greater than ten is your primary constitution.			
***Vikriti.* My Current State of Imbalance** If the grand total shows a humor more than forty from the sum of Parts I and II, this indicates an imbalance.			

APPENDIX II
The Concept of Six Tastes

Nature has packaged all possible food sources in to six tastes. Before the discovery of proteins, carbohydrates, fats, minerals, vitamins, and trace elements. Ayurveda believed that if we have all the six tastes in each of our meals, then we will have a balanced meal. The following lists are examples and not conclusive.

Sweet is a Vata- and Pitta-pacifying taste.
A sampling of the sweet foods includes:
* Most grains like wheat, rice, barley, corn, and most bread.
* Most legumes, such as beans, lentils, and peas.
* Milk and sweet milk products, such as cream, butter, and ghee.
* Sweet fruits like dates, figs, grapes, pears, and mangoes.
* Certain cooked vegetables, potatoes, sweet potatoes, carrots, and beets.
* All cooking oils including ghee, olive oil, coconut oil, sesame oil, and butter.
* Almonds, walnuts, pistachios, sunflower seeds, and nut milks.
* Sugar in any form, though not honey, which is considered astringent.

Sour is a Vata-pacifying taste.
A sampling of the sour foods includes:
* Sour fruits like lemon, lime, and sour oranges.
* Sour milk products like yogurt, cheese, sour cream, and whey.
* Fermented substances like wine, vinegar, soy sauce, and sour cabbage.

Salty is a Vata-pacifying taste.

A sampling of the salty foods includes:

❀ Any kind of salt.

❀ Foods to which a large amount of salt is added.

❀ Most sea vegetables and animals.

Pungent is a Kapha-pacifying taste.

A sampling of the heating-pungent foods includes:

❀ Spices like chili, black pepper, mustard seeds, ginger, cumin, and garlic.

❀ Certain vegetables, like radish and onion.

A sampling of the cooling-pungent foods includes:

❀ Spices, including coriander, fennel, basil, and dill.

Bitter is a Pitta- and Kapha-pacifying taste.

A sampling of the bitter foods includes:

❀ Certain fruits, like olives and grapefruits.

❀ Green, leafy vegetables like spinach, green cabbage, Brussels sprouts, and zucchini.

❀ Eggplant, bitter gourd, chicory, chocolate, and coffee.

❀ Certain spices, like turmeric and fenugreek.

Astringent is a Pitta- and Kapha-pacifying taste.

A sampling of the astringent foods includes:

❀ Legumes, beans, and lentils.

❀ Walnuts, hazelnuts, cashews, and pumpkin seed.

❀ Honey and black, green, and white teas.

❀ Sprouts, lettuce, and other green leafy vegetables; rhubarb; and most raw vegetables.

APPENDIX III

Create a Delicious Khichri of Mung Dal and Rice
Serves 4 - 5

6 cups water
8 oz. mung dal (split and peeled mung beans can be found online and at Indian stores)
4 oz. rice (the variety can be any; we recommend organic Jasmine, either white or brown)
2 bay leaves
1 heaping tbsp. ghee (vegans can substitute 1 Tbsp. organic unfiltered sesame or coconut oil)
1 tbsp. Mustard seeds (black or brown)
1 tbsp. Cumin seeds
Pinch of hing (also called asafoetida)
1 heaping tsp. turmeric powder
1 level tsp. ground black pepper
1 tsp. ground coriander seeds
6-10 pods cardamom
1 heaping tbsp. fresh ginger root, washed, peeled, and finely grated
2 tbsp. fresh lime or lemon juice
4 tbsp. fresh cilantro, roughly chopped, divided in half
1 tsp. powdered Himalayan sea salt
3 ½ Cups Raw dark leafy greens, like bok choy, kale, or spinach, chopped
  *A note on the spices: if there are additional tastes you crave or like, try them out in the recipe. This is a dish that can be created with

many flavor profiles. We each have our favorites. Ambika always adds cinnamon.

Stovetop Cooking Instructions

Rinse mung dal and rice and place them in a large cooking pot with the water and bay leaves. Cover and bring to a boil.

Reduce the heat and stir every 15 minutes as it simmers on medium-low heat until the mixture is soft—about 45 minutes to 1 hour.

While the mixture is cooking and you are visiting to stir it, you will notice frothy foam on the surface. Use a spoon to remove this foam from top of the mixture and discard it.

Pressure-Cooker Cooking Instructions

Place the mung, rice and bay leaves in the pressure cooker. Lock the lid down and bring to temperature on medium-high heat. Allow the whistle to blow two times.

Turn the heat down for approximately 10 to 12 minutes.

Turn the heat off. Let the pot sit for another 20 minutes without heat.

Open by running cold water over top of pot in sink to reduce pressure, and then set aside.

While the Mung and Rice Are Cooking Create a Vagar or Tadka, the Tempering of Spices in Hot Oil

Place the ghee or oil in an iron sauté pan and warm to a medium heat.

Add the cumin and mustard seeds. When the seeds begin to pop, the Vagar is sufficiently heated.

Add the turmeric powder, black pepper, ground coriander seeds, cardamom pods and grated ginger root. Let the spices marry with the oil and become irresistibly fragrant.

Add a cup or so of cooked mung and rice to the Vagar. Stir them together and then spoon it back into the original pot with the mung and rice. Use a little warm drinking water to get the last bit of Vagar out of the pan. Stir the mixture well to incorporate the spices.

To Serve

Mix in the fresh lemon or lime juice and half of the cilantro.

Use the remaining cilantro as a fresh garnish.

Serve with a side of your favorite chopped and lightly steamed vegetable. Be sure to heat the greens only until they are vibrant in color. This takes seconds. A good way to prevent overcooking is to heat the water and add the fresh chopped greens once it is up to temperature. Remove and add to the plate immediately.

Before Enjoying

Take a moment and give thanks for all the hands that brought this food to you—from seed and planting to harvest and store. Give gratitude for being able to create the meal and bless your food. This infuses the meal with love that will permeate your body with happiness.

APPENDIX IV
Self-Massage

Massaging your body with oil is an important aspect of the daily routine that provides a stabilizing influence all year long. Massage nourishes the tissues, stimulates the skin to release health-promoting chemicals, improves the circulation, increases alertness, facilitates detoxification, and improves immunity.

The purpose of the Ayurvedic daily massage as part of the daily routine is to prevent the accumulation of physiological imbalances and to lubricate and promote flexibility of the muscles, tissues, and joints. The classical texts of Ayurveda indicate that daily massage rejuvenates the skin and promotes youthfulness.

Choosing and Curing the Oil
Sesame oil is used unless a specific oil blend has been recommended, as it settles all three Doshas. If you find sesame oil unsuitable in some way, we recommend you try olive oil or coconut oil as an alternative.

❂ Please be aware that oils are highly flammable, for this reason they should be cured in the following way:
  ❀ Always warm them on a low setting.
  ❀ Never leave oil unattended.
  ❀ Once the oil reaches the proper temperature, remove it from the heat source and store it in a safe place until it cools.

How to Do Your Daily Massage

❋ Warm 1/4 cup of cured oil to slightly above body temperature. Place small amount of the oil on the fingertips and palms and massage vigorously using the open part of the hands rather than the fingertips.

❋ Begin by massaging the head. Cover the entire scalp with small circular strokes using the fingertips. The head is said to be one of the most important parts to emphasize during the daily massage.

❋ Next apply oil gently with the open part of the hand to your face and outer part of your ears. You can be gentle with these areas.

❋ Massage all areas of the neck and the upper part of the spine. Continue to use your open hand in a rubbing motion.

❋ Next apply a small amount of oil to each area of the body— head, face, arms, chest and abdomen, back and spine, legs, and feet. By focusing on smaller areas at a time, you are able to have maximum contact with a greater portion of the body.

❋ Massage your arms. The proper motion is up and down in the direction of the long bones of the limbs. Continue with circular motion over the joints. Massage both arms, including the hands and fingers.

❋ Next apply oil to the chest and abdomen. A very gentle circular motion is used over your heart. Use a gentle circular motion over the abdomen as well. Ayurveda traditionally advises moving in a clockwise direction. A straight up-and-down motion is used over the center of the chest and breast bone.

❋ Massage the back and spine, reaching whatever areas you can without straining.

❋ Massage the legs. Just as you did with the arms, use a long motion following the long bones of the limbs and a circular motion over the joints.

❋ Lastly, massage the bottom of the feet. The feet are considered especially important, and it is recommended that you spend more time here than on other parts of the body. Use the open part of your hands and massage vigorously back and forth over the sole of the foot.

Washing the Oil Off

Wash yourself with warm—not hot—water and mild soap. This helps to keep a small undetectable film of oil on the body after the bath, which is considered beneficial.

Ideally, about ten to twenty minutes should be spent each morning on the massage. However, if this time is not available on a particular day, it is better to do a brief massage rather than to skip the massage altogether. The most important parts to cover are the head and feet.

WHAT PEOPLE ARE SAYING ABOUT UNFOLDING HAPPINESS

"Our natural state of bliss is obscured by our thoughts, feelings, emotions, judgment, criticism, likes, dislikes, and trauma. That's why people are suffering. This book brings a practical approach to unfolding inner happiness and joy through a clinical approach to Ayurveda. It is a helpful guide to every Ayurvedic individual who seeks happiness."

Vasant Lad, BAM&S, MASc, Ayurvedic Physician
Author of *Ayurveda: Science of Self-Healing: A Practical Guide* and *Textbook of Ayurveda*

"Happiness resides within us, but we have forgotten how to access it and instead run after all the new gadgets and glitter of information technology. Dr. Vijay Jain unfolds the yogic secrets of uncompromised and unshakeable peace and happiness so that we can move beyond all dependencies and additions. His book makes for fascinating reading, providing many practical tools and transformative insights as how to discover the Ananda, or bliss, that is our true immortal nature."

Dr. David Frawley, Director, American Institute of Vedic Studies
Teacher of Yoga, Ayurveda, and Jyotish
Padma Bhushan Awardee
Author of *Shiva, the Lord of Yoga* and over thirty other books

"Happiness is our true nature, but the ego-mind hides this with attachments, aversions, and emotions, which create illness and depression. Ambika and Vijay reveal the insightful ancient teachings of yogic and Ayurvedic lifestyle that removes the obstacles to inner happiness, performing miracles in healing. Through their knowledge and inspiring personal stories you will learn how to provide the right conditions to naturally unfold into the state of happiness. This book will touch your heart and transform your life."

Yogi Amrit Desai, International Yoga Grand Master
Founder of Kripalu Yoga and Spiritual Leader of the Amrit Yoga Institute

"Unfolding Happiness is an extraordinary book—a beautiful rendering of ancient wisdom updated through a modern lens. The authors are well-versed in the subject, yet the book is far from a dry exposition. The authors have effectively woven personal stories and practical tips into every chapter, taking readers on a journey towards unfolding happiness. No matter where you are in your life, there is a gift for you in these pages."

Susan S. Freeman, Founder and President of "Step Up Leader," Author, and Speaker

"Enjoyable and interactive, Unfolding Happiness illustrates and reveals the possibility of living life as a joyous celebration through communicating with readers. The Sanskrit glossary, with simple translations, enhances the usability of the book for Ayurveda and Yoga readers seeking health as the foundation of happiness."

Dr. B.V.K. Sastry, Yoga-Samskrutham University

"Ambika and Vijay keep it REAL! Their heartfelt stories about the small victories and the pursuit of happiness hit just the right spot."

Dave Romanelli, Author of *Happy is the New Healthy*

"When I think about happiness now, after recently reading the intriguing words of Unfolding Happiness by Ambika Devi and Dr. Vijay Jain, new ideas on the subject float through my mind like kites or party balloons, or confetti in a parade. They urge me on to explore, ruminate, play, and luxuriate in the fantastic plethora of newfound wisdom they offer that wafts up in a fantastical celebration of frontal cortex enlightenment and bliss. This is not the usual tired, recycled wisdom one typically encounters in similar books of this genre. As you might guess, I can't recommend this book highly enough, and sincerely thank the authors for such a thoughtful and insightful analysis of all that happiness means in our individual voyages through life."

Dr. Patagonia, poet

More literary brilliance
from Mythologem Press!

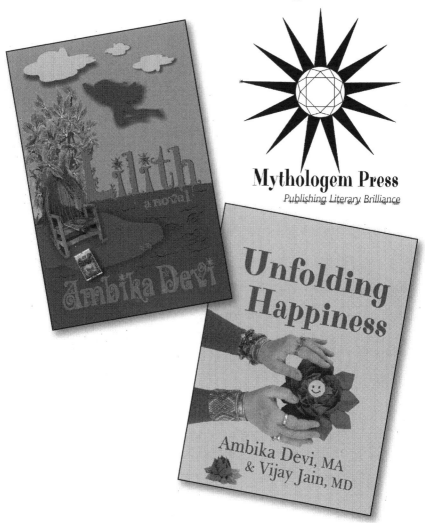

Mythologem Press
Publishing Literary Brilliance

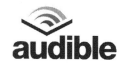

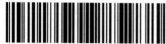

Made in the USA
Columbia, SC
10 June 2018